Evelin Kirkilionis

A Baby Wants to be Carried

Evelin Kirkilionis

A Baby Wants

to be Carried

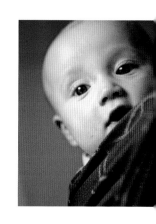

Everything you need to know about baby carriers and the benefits of babywearing

With photographs by Susanne Krauss

Throughout this book, the baby or child is referred to as 'he' to avoid burdening the reader repeatedly with phrases such as 'he or she', 'his or her' and so on. All references to a male baby or child therefore apply equally to a female baby or child.

A Baby Wants to be Carried

This first English-language edition published by Pinter & Martin Ltd 2014

Original title: *Ein Baby will getragen sein. Alles über geeignete Tragehilfen und die Vorteile des Tragens* by Evelin Kirkilionis

© 1999/2013 Kösel-Verlag, a division of Verlagsgruppe Random House GmbH, München, Germany.

ISBN 978-1-78066-145-2

The right of Evelin Kirkilionis to be identified as the author of this work have been asserted by her in accordance with the Copyright, Designs and Patent Act of 1988.

Cover: Susanne Krauss

Illustrations: Mascha Greune

Editor: Katrin Fischotter

Translated by: Kathryn O'Donoghue

Index: Helen Bilton

Layout: Karin Fercher

British Library Cataloguing-in-Publication Data
A catalogue record for this book is available from the British Library.

Printed in the EU by Hussar Books

Pinter & Martin Ltd
6 Effra Parade
London SW2 1PS

www.pinterandmartin.com

Contents

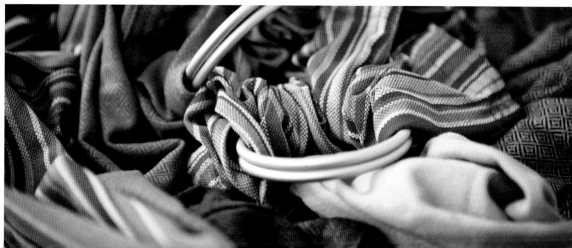

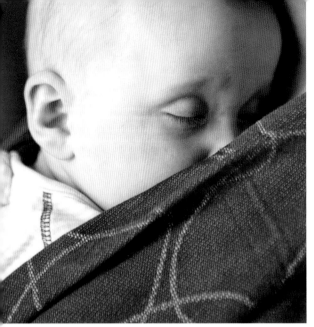

Introduction

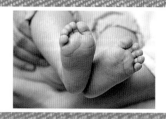

Nowadays, it has become commonplace to see a baby in a sling, wrap or carrier with buckles or straps. The benefits of transporting children this way, often known as 'babywearing', are undeniable. You can stride up and down stairs, go on a long walk in the countryside, or take a relaxed stroll through the market crowds without continually saying 'Excuse me, could I get through?' as you receive hostile looks when the pushchair ploughs through the crowd, stopping and starting. You don't feel like an obstacle when getting onto the bus and there are no wheels to lock with those of other pushchairs on a crowded train. Many minor or major everyday problems are easier to manage. For some mothers, carrying their children becomes a genuine survival strategy that goes some way towards helping them manage daily challenges. After all, looking after a baby is not the only thing that has to be tackled in family life, although for a single person it is often a full-time job on its own.

There's also the cosy feeling of closeness – on both sides. By keeping your child close to your body, you can feel his warmth and his every movement, and also directly feel his current condition. And the little one feels comfortable being so close to the 'source of his security'. He may hardly make a sound; as soon as you have gone down the steps into the fresh air, he may give just a contented grunt that sounds a little like 'Ah, finally,' before he contentedly falls asleep.

Of course, physical contact and closeness are important for an infant, but is all this focus on it a fuss about nothing? After all, for decades children have grown up using pushchairs and they have turned out OK – haven't they? Even so, many midwives and health professionals emphasise how important physical contact is and enthuse about slings or wraps in which the child sits nestled at the front. Those made from a large piece of material, which is wrapped around and around like a sarong worn in more temperate climates, looks rather tricky. A compact soft structured carrier would probably be better, but there are varied opinions on these. And to be upright straight from birth – is that even a good thing? Perhaps it would be better at the start to try a cradle carry with all this fabric – but what's the right way to do it? And when can I carry my baby in such and such a way without doing anything wrong?

Conflicting feelings and opinions, question after question – how, from when, and even why – have accompanied the issue of babywearing since this method became part of modern childcare. Nevertheless, babywearing has cast off the aura of being an 'alternative' to conventional pushchair use, and today slings, wraps and other carriers are available in almost every baby equipment shop. However, this rediscovered method of childcare and child transport – which is also an ancient part of our own culture – is still widely discussed.

Many of the same concerns as twenty years ago continue to unsettle parents thinking about carrying their child, or even stop them from doing so altogether. Questions relating to the supply of oxygen to the little one and the question of whether the spine is under too much pressure are common. Grandparents say it will spoil the child, and the scepticism of some paediatricians and physiotherapists is undiminished. If a complete stranger asks you which 'faith' you belong to, you may find it amusing.[1] But an aggressive question, like: 'Do you know what you are doing to your child?' is much less welcome.

Of course, parents also receive positive responses to babywearing. However, even though carrying babies has shed its exotic connotations and more and more young

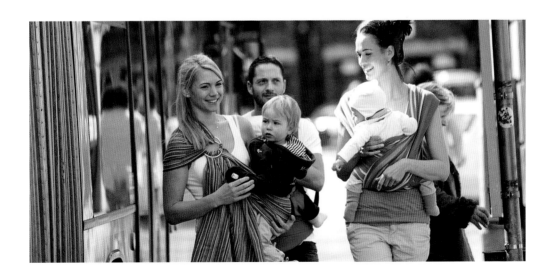

mothers are flirting with this form of childcare, there are still some reservations. Only proven background knowledge helps with uncertainties of this type. Even if practical tips on carrying are important, they are not the focus of this book, although they take up a lot of the pages. After all, nowadays, competent advice on tying techniques and carrying options is available in more and more countries. Sometimes midwives give courses and advice on how to carry a baby correctly and there are trained consultants, competent baby-wearing experts and even classes to teach you how to carry a baby. Sometimes the manufacturers of slings and

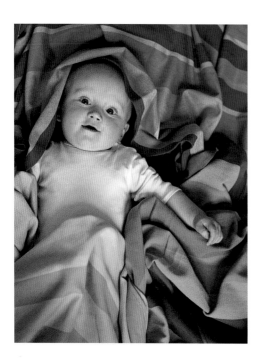

wraps offer their own courses; and illustrated descriptions of the different tying techniques are provided with every product or made available on the internet. You can browse through hundreds of websites for days on end and see the different tying methods presented in videos – some of which are more professional than others. The enthusiasm for experimentation by fans of babywearing has brought a flood of diverse carrying options – some of which unfortunately are unsuitable. If they were all to be mentioned, they would exceed the scope of this book. However, I introduce the basic tying methods and highlight the critical points to draw attention to questionable and unsuitable carrying methods. This will help you to reject them and avoid making mistakes.

It is also a particular concern of this book to awaken your understanding of the basic needs of a child, which are founded in our evolutionary history. I will introduce you briefly to the intellectual world of evolution and also examine anatomical features from biological and medical perspectives. Here you will also find supporting arguments to establish how topical and – hopefully – interesting evolutionary history and even anatomy can be. Both form the background to our understanding of the basic needs and behaviour of an infant. The understanding that many parents have unconsciously or intuitively plays an important role in the successful emotional relationship between the young and adult participants. More than anything else, parents at the start of a good parent–child relationship need to be sensitive to the behaviour of the baby, whose room for manoeuvre is initially restricted. Even if a baby is nowadays no longer regarded as a helpless bundle of reflexes and could provide adequate scientific proof of his abilities, he still won't be able to cope with circumstances or interactions that are not appropriate for his stage of development. This is where the parents come in. They not only satisfy the baby's needs and help him to develop the feeling of inner security that is so important for development, but they are also responsible for setting the framework in which a baby can assert and develop his abilities. Thus it is the parents who must initially provide a suitable environment – and they are generally able to do this. Unfortunately, however, circumstances sometimes prevent it and parents then need support and help in looking after the baby. All these issues are connected to babywearing, which is far more than just a convenient form of transport.

Wrap; woven wrap	Woven wraps are made out of specially manufactured material and come in a wide variety of lengths and colours. Rebozo are small wraps originating in South America, often made out of synthetic textile fibre. Stretchy wraps are made with the addition of Lycra/Spandex and are used for newborns and young babies.
Sling	Often used synonymously for wraps. Sometimes used only for wrap-like carriers like pouches (see page 166), ring slings (see page 165), etc.
Asian-style carrier	Mei Tai, Onbuhimo, podegai etc. have long straps that have to be tied.
Soft structured carrier (SSC)/ full buckle	Carriers with padding which are adjustable with straps and buckles. Many carriers available in popular brands on the high-street need careful investigation before purchase to make sure the baby is properly supported and the parent's back will not suffer (see page 108). There are, however, good-quality highly supportive brands on the market too.
Half buckle	Asian style carrier with a plastic buckle at the waist and long shoulder straps which are tied like a wrap.
Wrap conversions	Carriers made out of wraps which may have buckles, wrap straps, padding or sling rings added. They are often created as customized works for individual customers.

Table 1 Types of babycarriers.

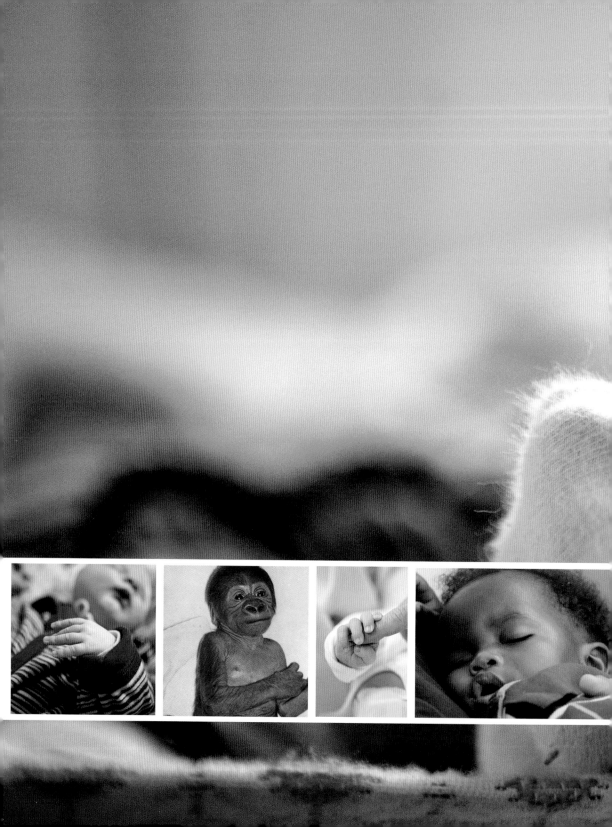

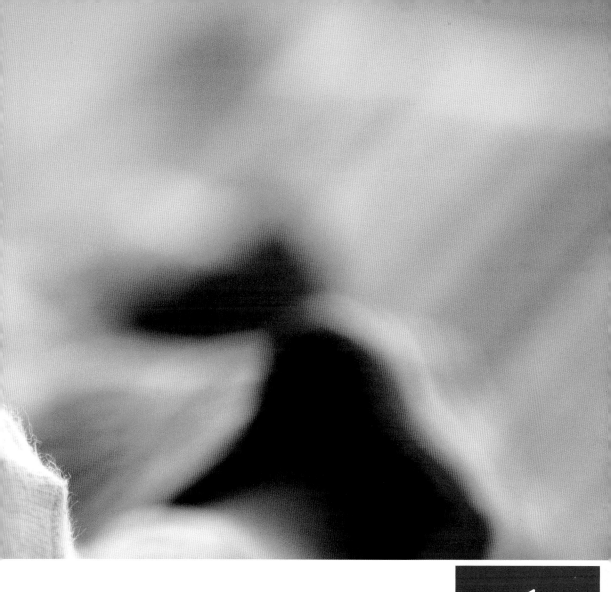

The theory of babywearing: why carry your child?

1

Closeness and Security

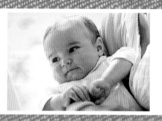

The need for closeness versus the fear of spoiling your child

'I don't know why but for a while now Nicholas just won't go to sleep. We even have a separate peaceful bedroom for him.' The words of the parents resound with surprise, disappointment and confusion. Previous living arrangements did not allow a separate children's bedroom. For the midday nap, the Moses basket was placed on the corner seat next to the kitchen table and, in spite of the couple's best efforts, most of the time it was quite noisy. However, usually the baby fell asleep straight away. And now there are difficulties trying to get him to sleep in his own, quiet, lovingly decorated bedroom. It seems that capricious demands are behind this. After all, a peaceful separate room creates the proper sleep environment for an adult. However, an infant has other needs. For him, absolute silence is far from the best

pre-requisite for sleep. Think about the baby who catnaps on his father's lap while the rest of the family chat loudly around the kitchen table; or the scene in which the little one peacefully falls asleep huddled in a sling or wrap on his mother while his siblings romp around the two of them with their friends. **It's not peace and quiet that he needs, it's the *calming* sense of the person providing security that is important to enable a baby to fall asleep.**

'You can't even go out of the room for a minute without her becoming unsettled or starting to cry. Anouk is already spoiled!' How many mothers have heard this comment or similar from the older generation? The idea of the egotistical infant who needs to be taught as early as possible that she shouldn't 'play up' seems impossible to eradicate.

Firstly, comments of this type *prevent* parents from following their initial impulse and picking up the baby, or in other words from yielding to their 'intuitive parenting skills'. Secondly, they also *prevent* parents from providing their child with calming closeness. This means that they are not meeting their child's basic needs.

The proximity of his parents gives a baby a sense of security, safety and peace – and this is true far beyond the age of infancy. Contact with familiar people is also the most important prerequisite for a child over the next few years to enable him to explore his environment in a balanced and enquiring way. Of course, over time, the child has more room for manoeuvre. At some point it will be enough for him to know that his parents are in the next room, simply to hear them, and now and then run to them and 'stock up' on their closeness. However, in distressing situations direct physical contact will still be necessary. But for now let us focus on infancy.

The above-mentioned concept of the 'basic need' has already been suggested: when demanding the proximity of a familiar person, biology plays an important role. An infant likes to have the people who care for him close by as much as possible. After all, a baby doesn't know that he is growing up in a protected environment, that – even when he is lying alone in his bed – there is no danger and he is no longer on the menu for cave bears and other wild animals. Whichever way we look at it: **the genetic features of our behaviour largely correspond to those of the hunter–gatherer societies of our evolutionary history, which only gradually disappeared with the first human settlements 10,000 years ago.** Of course, as part of our individual development we learn that this is no longer the case. This ability to learn is also embedded in our genetic make-up and makes humans the 'evolutionary model of success' they have proven to be. Such spiritual creativity enables a human to react to the changing conditions of life. However, the younger and less experienced a person, the stronger the pull of the innate components of his

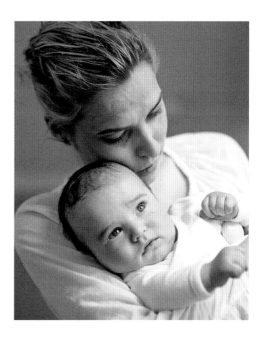

Intuitive parenting

Parents and any adults receptive to a child's signals unconsciously notice how the infant is feeling and react intuitively to them – and, for the most part, do so in a manner appropriate to their situation and abilities. Even without any experience, this intuitive parenting can enable anyone who is receptive to the signals of a child to interact effectively with them. However, it is important that nothing unsettling, disturbing or stressful masks the intuitive parenting. This is because although intuitive parenting has a biological basis, it is susceptible to interference. In some cases intuitive parenting cannot overcome the current conditions and is quickly masked or suppressed, particularly by stress.

Intuitive parenting can be seen, for example, when parents unconsciously speak to their baby in a higher tone of voice, slowly, and with overemphasis: they modify their behaviour to match the baby's ability, using repetition and adjusted speech rhythm. This 'baby talk' is accompanied by overemphasised, slower facial expressions. The reactions to the signals of the child are precisely tailored to the baby, as is the distance of the parent's face to the child. This is because babies are short-sighted at first and their optimum viewing range is 20 to 25cm (8 to 10in). Parents subconsciously perceive this and always move into the correct position to catch the baby's attention and thus keep in contact.

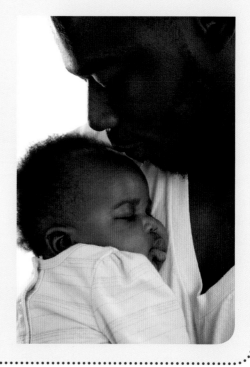

behaviour, and he must thus focus more closely on the framework conditions. This primordial behaviour 'says' to a baby: 'Look, the people who protect you from the dangers in the world are always around you! They are the only ones who will give you everything you need, who mean security, who guarantee your survival and who will keep wolf and co. in check!'

If we broadly consider the way of life of our human ancestors, from the very start the history of humankind was shaped by the permanent mobility of the entire group, which was required for gathering food and hunting. This was the norm for a period of around five million years – except for during the most recent 10,000 years during which humans gradually settled down. Because of the nomadic way of life throughout most of human evolutionary history, offspring were genetically predisposed to be carried and were breastfed frequently. Our closest relations, for example chimpanzees, still demonstrate this behaviour today. And our babies are still 'programmed' to expect to be handled in a similar way. **According to a baby's biological programming, to stay somewhere alone means only one thing – not only being left behind by the person caring for him, but also being *abandoned*, or in other words finding himself in mortal danger.** With this evolutionary background, it logically follows that a baby left alone in a room or in his cot to sleep would immediately become unsettled. As a result – if his initial contact signals are not answered – he will try with all his strength to call for the person providing protection.[2] He initially has only a few methods at his disposal. Loud crying is the most effective and this normally also fulfils the purpose. Even total strangers are startled by the crying and feel the need to look after the 'poor baby', to pick him up, rock him and soothe him when they hear the dramatic cries of abandonment. This is where behavioural biology shows itself – even with adults who are actually not involved – as the intuitive parenting programme is not restricted to parents, but exists in all adults.

Our evolutionary history actually overrides the 'spoiling' argument – at least in terms of suckling infants. However, if you don't want to grapple with our evolution at this point, there is another important argument to consider: the cognitive limits of a child of this age.

An infant lives in the here and now, and objects, and of course also people, only exist if they can be directly perceived by him. **It is not until the baby is around nine months old that objects and people continue to exist for him even if he can't see, hear or touch them.** Babies already

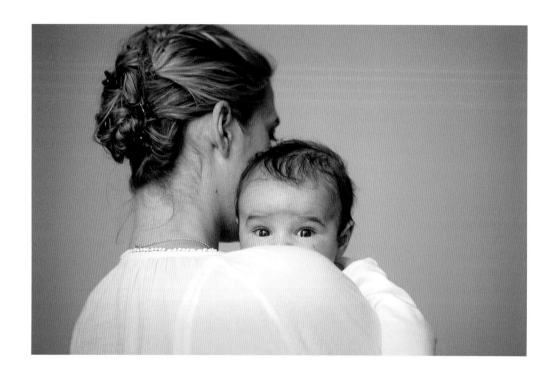

have the rudiments of this 'object permanence' in the fifth to sixth month of life, but not until three to four months later do they actively seek out the object that has disappeared from their field of vision.[3] Thus, in the early months, an infant can't be sure of the continued existence of his parents and, consequently, of their care, when they have disappeared from his field of vision. Against the background of the child's abilities it is thus completely logical that when a baby is laid down in a separate room, he can't fall asleep. Even as adults we can usually only fall straight asleep when nothing is troubling us and our world has been put to rights. **The baby's world, however, has not been put to rights if the parents who protect and thus calm him are absent or he can't sense them in any way.** In this situation, the reaction is pure stress resulting from fear. Even for an older child, it is not always easy to fall asleep alone. This is a skill that needs to be learnt. Is it reasonable that we sometimes demand something from a baby of just a few months old that is difficult even for adults: to find peace in a stressful situation?

Given the above, the fact that the need for security is particularly strong when going to sleep is hardly surprising. However, nor is it always the case that a baby in a sling or a wrap immediately falls asleep, as some mothers find to their surprise during their first experience of using one: 'During that time, he never slept.' There is hardly a better recipe for finding peace and taking a nap than to be cuddled up in physical contact with mum or dad, especially when the rocking movement starts with every step.

The desire for constant closeness and physical contact is a basic need during babyhood. It is not until the baby is around nine months old that objects and people continue to exist for him even if he can't see, hear or touch them. Only then are the foundations laid for the child to understand that parental care continues even in their absence.

The clinging young – a quick course

Traditional cradles are actually nothing more than simulations of the parent moving. The fact that rocking is such an effective means of bringing calm is due to living conditions during our evolutionary history. As mentioned before, because of the nomadic life of early humans, offspring had to be carried. During long forays to find seasonal foods, babies spent most of the early part of their lives being carried close to the body of the mother or an accompanying trusted person. However, it doesn't do justice to the significance of this adaptation to restrict it to the hunter–gatherer period of human evolution. One reason for this is that traditional cultures that live as hunter–gatherers still exist today, and they can thus give us an idea of how our ancestors lived. Even our upright walking 'prehuman' ancestors – possibly *Australopithecus* means something to you – can be included in this analysis. In this early evolutionary period the young would still have been carried on the mother's body. Thus we can readily speak of a 'carrying tradition' founded in the evolutionary history of around four to six million years ago (scientists continue to argue about the exact age of the first findings relating to the ancestors of humans). Human infants of today,

concerned with their current needs, have therefore been generally predisposed since the beginning of the history of humankind to be constantly in direct contact with one of their caregivers during the early stages of life, which means they 'expect' to be carried by those caregivers. If we include our early non-human ancestors in this history, and if we don't shrink away from a look at the animal species most closely related to us, (such as the different types of monkeys and apes, who display similar carrying behaviour), we can find **a genetic predisposition to being carried that goes back 55 million years.**[4] (For more on this, see page 24). In contrast, there is a period of a paltry 10,000 years after this, during which groups of humans began to settle in communities where their offspring could be put down in a safe place. In terms of the span of evolution of humans, this recent period of time is too short for the infant's behaviour to have adapted to the safe environment.

In addition to these findings from evolutionary history, various behavioural, anatomical and physiological facts prove that a baby is predisposed to expect to be carried. These range from the grip reflex of the hands and feet, to the spread–squat reaction, to the prophylaxis against hip dysplasia (more on this on page 42 onwards). If you want to look at this subject in more detail, in-depth questions and answers are included in the next chapter. At this point, I would like to re-emphasise the following points. Today, as before, an infant is predisposed to be carried, just like his newborn *Australopithecus* ancestor; and, as before, his needs are focussed on this; also, as before, he still counts as 'clinging young', a description that takes into account his behaviour in the first year of life. This concept is representative of the different behavioural traits of a newborn, including his emotional needs, which can be regarded as an important achievement of adaptation. In evolutionary prehistoric times, they guaranteed survival and thus also the survival of the human race.

This evolutionary excursion clarifies why carrying our babies has such a calming effect on them and shows how evolutionary

Traditional cultures – a window into the past

Traditional cultures are generally societies living in small groups, that are scarcely or not at all influenced by the technical/civilised world, i.e. they generally live close to nature. 'Palaeolithic' hunter–gatherer cultures and/or hunters or 'Neolithic' horticulturists originally used only stones, bones, wood etc. for producing utensils. They can be considered an 'ideal model' for the various early stages in the development of human culture.

Some examples of hunter–gatherer societies are the South African !Kung or the East African Hadza. They give us an idea of the social relationships and how people lived in the hunter–gatherer stage of evolutionary history. From this stage we have inherited most of our genetically conditioned behaviours. Around 10,000 years ago, humans began to give up their hunter life-style and became settled. This is too short a time for changes in behavioural patterns determined by our genes to have taken place. Thus people of today are also predisposed to living in small groups of between 40 and a maximum of 150 people, subdivided into small family units. Communities did not evolve into larger, more complex societies until around 6,000 years ago.[5]

Types of young: altricial, precocial and clinging young

In biology, the young of different mammalian species are classified into three types according to their developmental stage and their behaviour after birth: altricial, precocial and clinging young.

Altricial (stay-at-home, or sometimes *nidiculous*): this includes young mice and rabbits, which are very immature when born. Their eyes and auditory canals are closed for protection; the more primordial and typical examples have no hair. Blind and hardly able to move, they spend their early life in the protection and warmth of the nest, where they are also often left alone by the mother for long periods. Later, when the young can move independently, they flee to the protective nest when there is danger.

Precocial (flee-the-nest, or sometimes *nidifugous*): examples are horse foals and elephant calves, which are relatively mature when born. To be able to follow the mother soon after the birth, their bodies must be physiologically well developed. Their sensory systems and temperature and motion controls must function immediately. These young thus have hair and show a wide range of behavioural patterns. Mother and young stay in constant contact with each other. It is striking that the unborn animal goes through a sort of 'altricial' phase within its mother's body, which means that its eyes and auditory canals close during foetal development but open again before birth. The precocial young type is thus derived from the altricial type, which was the more ancestral type for mammals.

The terms nidiculous or nidifugous are sometimes used, but their meaning differs slightly. Altricial and precocial refer to the stage of development, while nidiculous and nidifugous describe whether the young leave or stay in the nest. Some nidiculous young are well developed and able to leave the nest, whereas nidifugous young are also precocial.

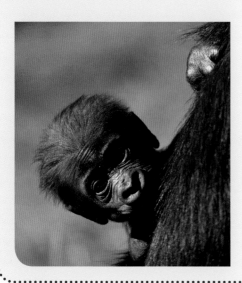

Active clinging young (sometimes referred to as *parent clingers*) are significantly more mature when they are born. Their eyes and auditory canals function after birth, and they close and open during foetal development. Thus they also derived from the altricial type, as they run through the 'altricial' phase in the uterus 'again' as per the evolutionary development. They are physiologically well-developed so that although they cannot move in the manner of their species immediately after birth, they can hold onto their mother's fur independently. Their first habitat is the mother's body. They have hair and can regulate their temperature through physical contact with the mother. They also show a wide range of behaviours. During their development, the protective 'place' remains the mother; the young also flee and return to the mother to escape danger later when they are capable of moving. *Passive clinging young* such as kangaroos – which I don't want to dwell on here – have a similar development status to the altricial young and spend their post-natal development in the mother animal's fold of skin or pouch.

history can be very interesting and up-to-date. It gives important insights into the patterns of life of our early ancestors, and can explain and help us to understand the sometimes puzzling behaviour of our infants today. It can also help you create an environment more suitable for your child.

In biological terms the human infant is an example of clinging young. His complete development and behaviour has been predisposed to this since the start of human evolutionary history, and is as valid today as in the past.

The human infant: a special case

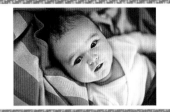

The clinging young – and its special history

If you want to further your knowledge of this subject after the short introduction to evolutionary history in the preceding chapter, you can find further discussion of the clinging young and the importance of our evolutionary history here.

The 'clinging young' was defined after the 'altricial' type and 'precocial' type (for more on this, see page 22). These three concepts are short formulae for the respective adaptations of the young of a species to the most diverse of living and care conditions, and this includes humans. The short formulae are not simply a result of biologists' enthusiasm for categorising. The concepts are connected to their very own care conditions for a species and the needs of the offspring during the initial stages of life, with characteristic anatomical and physiological features and accompanying innate behavioural complexes.

The behavioural dispositions, our evolutionary history and comparisons with our closest relatives, the apes, clearly show that human newborns belong to the biological offspring type of clinging young. Clinging young are predisposed to being constantly carried. Active clinging young hold onto the mother independently. The offspring of different apes and, in particular, the great apes, hold on to the belly fur of the mother using their hands and feet. Later they often switch to a riding position.

However, the human infant cannot hold on to its mother's body with its hands and feet. We don't have fur any more, so our little ones have no chance of holding on to mummy. Also over time we have developed 'walking feet', and they can no longer grip well enough for secure clinging on. A baby's hand alone would not be strong enough for a secure hold, although in the first weeks of life the palmar grasp reflex of the hands and the plantar reflex of the feet is reminiscent of this ability from the early days of evolution. Maybe you are now thinking of the pictures of babies clinging to the washing line with their hands, who (understandably) don't look very happy. These are snapshots taken soon after birth. They are mostly low-weight, and often even premature babies. After a short time, the strength of the little one is no longer sufficient for such acrobatics. Although a human baby cannot hold on with either feet or hands, should it still be classed as clinging young and, if so, should it be an active one?

For the final explanation of this question, we must look again at our evolutionary history. Effective upright walking is inevitable with the transmutation of the lower limbs into walking feet which have a significantly restricted ability to grip. Even little *Australopithecus* had to battle this 'problem', right at the start of our human evolution. He could not hold on to the hair coat of his mother as effectively with his lower extremities either, unlike his closest relatives at that time who can still do so today.

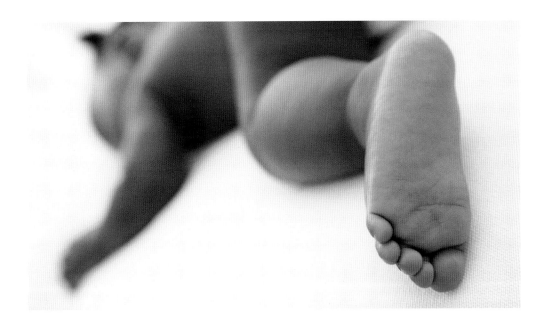

Australopithecus news: little Lucy was already standing upright

To the best of our current knowledge, the first representatives of the *Homo* genus come from one of the *Australopithecus* species. The *Homo* genus is the one to which modern man and our closest relatives such as the Neanderthals, who have since died out, belong; hence *Homo neanderthalensis, Homo habilis, Homo erectus* and others. Various species of *Australopithecus* walked upright and roamed through the East African savannah. Lucy (*Australopithecus afarensis*) and the child of Taung (*Australopithecus africanus*) became well-known. However, fossilised footprints were also exciting finds, as they proved the bipedal way of moving (this means upright, 'two-legged' walking) of these early pre-human species. The age estimates of the *Australopithecus* and *Homo* species have undergone radical revision many times in recent decades. Nowadays, a number of scientists tend to give younger age estimates. The start of the evolutionary history of humankind is taken from the point when the ancestors of humans diverged from that ancestor-population they shared with chimpanzee, and this is given in the available literature as 7.5 million years ago, as 6.3 to 5.4 million years ago, and as 6.3 to 4.1 million years ago. Nevertheless, today we can, in good conscience, estimate that the need to be carried has existed for approximately 6 million years. If we include our great ape ancestors, we get a figure of 20 to 22 million years; and if we add in the ape species, we get, as mentioned before, a 'carrying tradition' through our entire line of ancestors of 55 million years.[6]

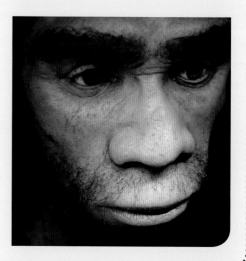

Little *Australopithecus* had already lost two of four grip and stabilisation points on his mother's body during this early period in evolutionary history. However, just like his ape-like relatives, he had to be carried constantly due to the unchanged mobile way of life and thus he undoubtedly belongs with the clinging young. To put it bluntly, the problem arose very early in the history of humankind and had to be solved just as early. With the great apes of today, the offspring are supported by the mother with a hand during the early days, although this significantly restricts their general ability to move. In fact, in critical situations, this can lead to a life-threatening situation for mother and child. Nevertheless it is conceivable that the *Australopithecus* mother provided greater support to her offspring. With the regression of the hair coat, the human mother had to take on the full carry load and, as a result, the infant became a passive clinging young. However, this would have been significantly restrictive to the actions of the mother and her freedom of movement; an extremely precarious development for the living conditions of that time.

In fact, in behavioural biology, the human infant was considered the passive clinging young type for many years. This doesn't take into account the resulting consequences for our earliest ancestors at the start of human evolutionary history, just like the human infant of today. Conversely, there are modes of behaviour and anatomical features that demonstrate the active participation of even the newborns of today in being carried. Expressed in layman's terms, little *Australopithecus*, or one of his descendants, introduced a unique carrying strategy: he looked for another place on the mother's body – the hip. Thus, with all the gradual changes in the course of human evolution – (the upright gait, accompanied by the physical modifications linked to the reshaping of the grasping, walking foot to a plain walking foot) – he could keep up without having to give up his status as active clinging young.

It is worth looking at this particular development in more detail as it still has consequences today. For a better understanding I would like to mention a few

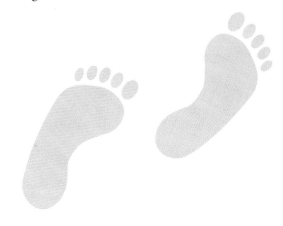

comparative observations. To prevent misunderstandings, I would also like to emphasise that the comparative approaches are only conceptual aids. Observations made of one animal species can never be simply transferred to other animal species, and therefore not to humans either – and vice versa. Species-specific investigations are always necessary.

Various elements accommodated this 'evolutionary slide' of the human infant to

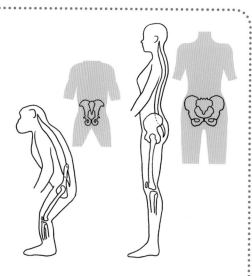

Fig. 1 Comparison of the upright body silhouettes of a human and chimpanzee. The shape of the pelvis and the spine are characteristic for the respective type of movement: upright on two legs/bipedal stature for the human, on hands and feet for chimpanzees (knuckle-walking posture).

the side and to the mother's hip. Firstly, the anatomical circumstances of the infant itself. The carrying mothers also play an important role. The skeletal adaptations to erect posture affected the whole of the skeleton of the pelvis, amongst other things.

Even in the large-scale illustration (see Fig. 1), the associated basic changes are easy to recognise. **In the mothers, this gives a distinct hip-waist area that accommodates the seat of the child on the hip – to be more precise, in the waist.** A wide pelvis with protruding ilia arched outwards, and a comparatively narrow waist gives a better hold to the mother's body than in the case of our closest relatives who lack a waist of this type. The silhouettes of the bodies also show this.

However, it is just as important that in our early history there were also pre-adaptations on the part of the child, which accommodated the new position on the mother's body. See the image of the gorilla baby as a conceptual aid (see Fig. 2, page 29). The spread, bent legs and the bent arms offer a good position for a small primeval gorilla, or indeed a modern one, to cling on in the mother's belly hair as soon as the opportunity arises. The soles of the feet are oriented more towards the front, as gorilla babies are carried to the front on the wide breast of the mother. This position is observed for all great ape offspring as soon as they are put down and it is highly probably that our early ape-like ancestors also behaved in this way.

This spread and squat leg posture is also a suitable starting position (see Fig. 3, below right) for a human child to hold on to the mother's body in a lateral hip carry: in fact, using his whole legs. A baby clasps the narrow side of the mother with tucked legs in the spread–squat position and stabilises his position by pressing with the upper and lower leg. With human babies it is striking that in the supine position, the soles of the feet are often oriented towards each other, useful in the hip carry (see Fig. 5, page 30) when the little feet could still grip. Sometimes, even today, babies touch loose folds of clothing with their toes, which is reminiscent of the plantar grasp reflex that was originally used to hold on to the coat, just like the palmar grasp reflex in the hands.

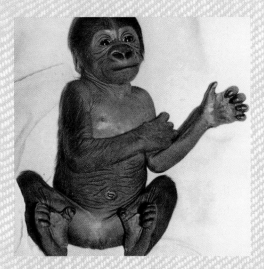

Fig. 2 The famous Basle gorilla baby Goma in the typical body posture of a young ape when it is put down.[7]

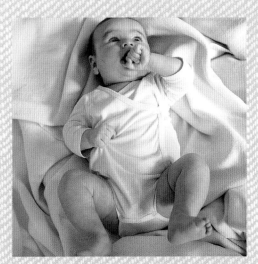

Fig. 3 An eleven-week-old baby seen here in a corresponding characteristic spread–squat posture (for more on this, see page 31).

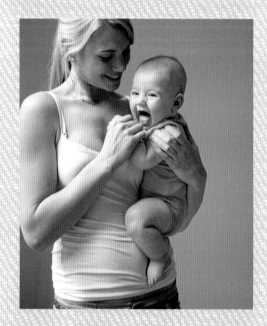

Fig. 4 Six-month-old baby in the hip carry position – the little legs grip the narrow side of the mother.

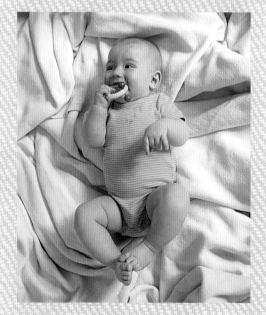

Fig. 5 A baby concentrates on a toy and 'incidentally' is also in the spread–squat position. The feet often face each other, reminiscent of the early period of evolutionary history when a baby could still hold onto the fur of the mother.

This spread–squat position shows that almost no changes or adjustments were necessary on the part of the infant in order to transfer the position on the mother's body from the front carrying method to the side. In biology, this is known as being 'pre-adapted'. This is almost a magical word in evolutionary biology, as pre-adaptations are prerequisites to enable changes to take place in the course of evolutionary history. The human infant is thus, as before, clinging young, however, with a specific development: He clings to the mother in a side hip carry in the spread-squat position. This position should be looked at for a number of different reasons.

Due to findings from evolutionary history and from comparing species, human infants are classified as active clinging young, with a unique development. Babies no longer hold onto the mother's body with their hands and feet like the closely related apes; instead they cling on in a side hip carry using their whole legs.

The innate behavioural patterns of modern human offspring

Following this quick tour of evolutionary history, let us now return to your baby, with his many little characteristics and, in particular, to the spread–squat position mentioned before. This position is uncomfortable and tiring for adults and requires willpower to hold for a long time. However, your baby likes to pull his legs up and part them slightly. The feet are often pointing towards or touching each other without being included in the moment's activities (see Figs. 3 and 5, pages 29 and 30). If this posture required conscious strength, a baby would not be able to hold this tiring position for a long time during an exploratory game as in Fig. 5, during which the baby is concentrating on a toy or deep in observation of an object. Certainly not for 20–30 minutes, as has been recorded in older babies of four to six months old. Some babies even fall asleep in this position. This leg posture must thus accommodate the anatomical and physiological conditions of an infant.[8] The process of movement of the six-month-old child when he is lifted from the ground (see Fig. 6a to c below), also highlights the connection between

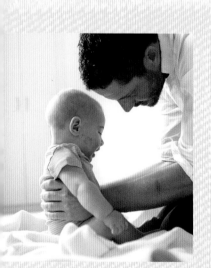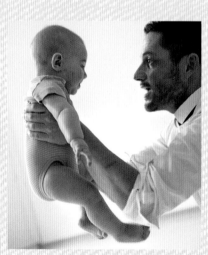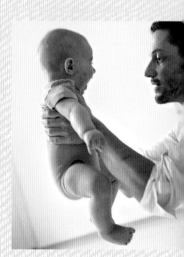

Fig. 6 a to c In expectation of being carried on the hip: the spread–squat reaction.

this body position and being carried. As soon as an infant loses contact with the ground, he pulls up the legs in this typical manner. In this strong bent posture with lightly spread legs, he can be easily placed on the hip. Babies regularly demonstrate this spread–squat reaction in the first weeks of life. When they are older, it tends to be only when they are accustomed to being carried – and when they expect this and also *want* this. Thus it is in no way a reflex reaction, as it is dependent on different factors. Just the fact that a baby is distracted by something interesting is enough to prevent this sequence of movements. It can therefore not be carried out at any moment (hence the expansion of the concept to reaction, not reflex). In particular, babies who are rarely carried, who are well padded with those cuddly chubby legs, show only a suggestion of this reaction. Here the force of gravity is the winner.

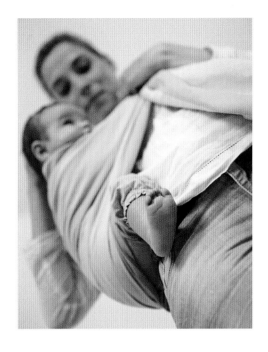

With this spontaneous leg position adopted when the baby is lifted up, he is actively preparing for the side hip carry. As a consequence, to be carried is by no means a passive event for a baby. The baby is also active during the hip carry. You can feel this when you move unexpectedly or sharply. In this case, the child presses his legs harder against your body. He grips tighter and actively stabilises his position, which is something that older children with more developed motor skills are able to do. Reactions of this type are, of course, dependent on the physical development of the infant. Babies of only a few weeks old tend to press their legs onto the mother rather then wrap them around. However, as their ability to control their body grows, they can hold on properly, even though they are dependent on the support of the carrying person. **So infants by no means play a passive role in being carried. They prepare for the hip carry position with the spread–squat reaction and even take part in the stabilisation of the position themselves.** In everyday life this doesn't mean that the dear little ones do not trustingly depend on mummy and daddy. They confidently leave the parent to take the strain while they loosely swing their legs to and fro and make little gymnastic movements – to recklessly test out the limits of the strength and reactions of their parental safety basis, in the truest sense of the word.

Human infants are unique in their behaviour as current and active clinging young and this is also supported by their anatomical features. In fact, even symptoms of illness prove that the status of clinging young is still valid today. And so we arrive at the topic of hip dysplasia; firstly however, let's look at the special anatomical features of the child, in particular the spine.

An infant is anatomically and physiologically disposed to being carried on the hip in a spread and squatting position. He actively prepares for the hip carry with the spread–squat reaction and also actively participates in the stabilisation of the hip carry position: He is still classed as active clinging young today.

The unique physiology and anatomy of newborn infants – the spine

The anatomical and physiological characteristics of the infant are modifications to the given conditions and specific demands of his early stages of life. They are clearly differentiated from those of adults. **The anatomy of a baby is initially not suitable for upright walking and the characteristics and function of the spine, pelvis and legs are suited to being carried.**

The spine of a newborn infant lacks the double S-curve that is typical of an adult and which, due to its shape, acts as a buffer for the impact caused by walking and running, significantly reducing the shocks to different parts of the body and, in particular, to the sensitive brain. In infancy, the spine is straighter and the body seems to be slightly rounded (kyphosis). This doesn't mean, however, that the spine of a baby is semi-circular. It is more that he lacks the particular areas that are responsible for the distinct double S-shape of the adult, just as initially infants lack the distinctive posterior muscles needed for walking. These aren't needed yet and they develop as soon as they are actually required.

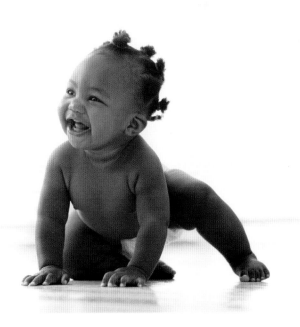

The spine of a newborn child – slightly rounded

The cervical and lumbar spines are almost straight in a newborn. The two areas that give an adult the typical slight double S-curve are missing (cervical and lumbar lordosis). The overall slightly rounded appearance of a child's back results firstly from the existing obvious kyphosis (curvature) in the thoracic vertebrae area and, secondly, from the lack of a distinct lordosis in the cervical area – which is characteristic of adults. As a result, the head and the shoulder area of a baby appear to fall forward. This impression is reinforced by a very narrow kink in the transition area between the lumbar spine region and the fused vertebrae of the sacrum, which are integrated into the pelvic girdle.[9] In adults, this gives the second S-curve the lumbar lordosis. The following figures may help to to present the significance of this situation better. In adults the promontory angle, which is related to this kink, is 60°, whereas in newborns it is only 20° (for comparison only – with chimpanzees it is 35°).[10] The spine of a newborn is thus by no means a semi-circle or round C, even though the torso appears overall to be kyphotic.

As soon as a baby lifts his head and finally begins to crawl, the previously nearly straight cervical spine starts to curve and cervical lordosis occurs. When the child begins to walk, the second S-curve of the spine will be gradually more and more formed: the lumbar lordosis. However, at the start, the gait of a child differs from that of an adult because the baby's spine and pelvis are still in a different position to each other (see also page 38). If the baby wants to walk forwards quickly, he doesn't put his heels down but instead first runs on his toes and the balls of his feet, as he cannot yet move his thighs very far backwards from the vertical body line. The final formation of the spine only takes place in puberty.

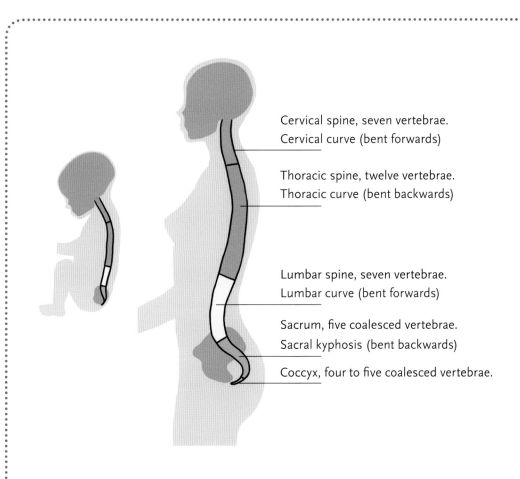

Cervical spine, seven vertebrae.
Cervical curve (bent forwards)

Thoracic spine, twelve vertebrae.
Thoracic curve (bent backwards)

Lumbar spine, seven vertebrae.
Lumbar curve (bent forwards)

Sacrum, five coalesced vertebrae.
Sacral kyphosis (bent backwards)

Coccyx, four to five coalesced vertebrae.

Fig. 7 Newborn spine compared with adult spine[11]

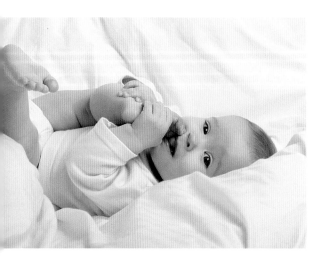

Consequently, during infancy the spine and pelvis have a different position to each other than in adulthood. If you draw a straight line through the torso and pelvis, the angle between both lines is narrower for the infant than for the adult. As a consequence of this, the hip joints in the pelvis are positioned further to the front. Adults can bend their legs but also move them far behind the vertical body line as is necessary for taking a long step. **In an infant, the hip joints are orientated further to the front, so the range of movement is restricted to the area in front of the body, a position that evolved to suit the living conditions of clinging young.**[12] Accordingly, when a baby is in a relaxed lying position, the legs fall outwards and, at the same time, they are slightly bent in the hip and knee areas. It would cause harm to an infant if the thighs and knees were pressed down properly onto the floor – i.e. if the baby were to lie like an adult with their legs stretched out. This would force the poor child to take evasive action: the pelvis would be tipped further 'forwards/down' and the spine would arch up and force the baby into a hollow back position, which conflicts with the physiological conditions for this age.

As a result of the lack of, or only slight, lordotic areas of a child's spine, the range of movement in an infant's leg is restricted to the area in front of the torso. This is a range of movement suitable for carrying. The torso appears slightly rounded as the lordosis in the cervical spine area is not yet distinct.

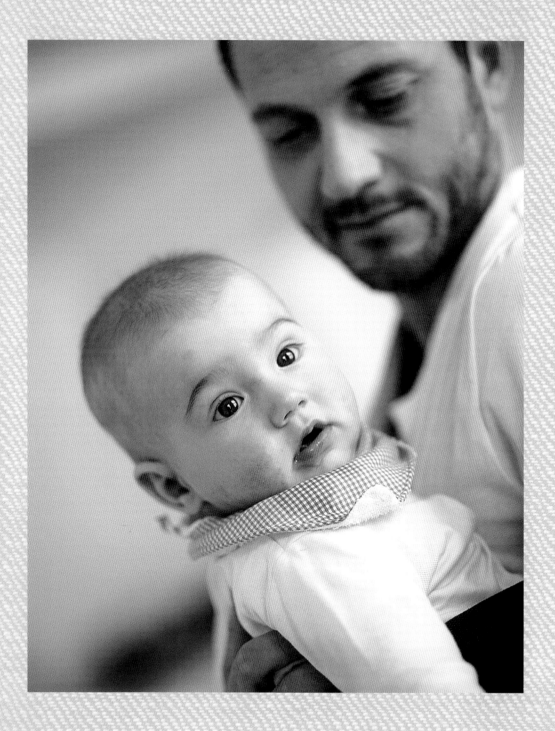

The unique physiology and anatomy of infants – the pelvis and hip joints

The position of the body and the extremities in infants, which appears bent compared to that of adults, caused doctors, wet nurses and mothers in different cultural groups to 'bandage' infants in early centuries. This was a type of swaddling, similar to the Native American papooses, in which the body and limbs were wrapped in long strips of cloth in a stretched, upright position so that in the future they would grow 'straight' and not be 'crooked' like a baby when adulthood was reached. However, these measures in no way supported a good upright posture or the health of children. Instead they encouraged congenital hip dysplasia and hip dislocation. Against the background of such hip-joint conditions, by 1961 the German orthopaedist Johannes Büschelberger had already had the idea of investigating the most anatomically favourable position of the femur and the femoral head in the hip-joint socket, using hip- joint specimens from newborns.[13] **He showed that the femoral head fits well inside the hip joint if the leg is tucked up and slightly spread.** To be specific, this means that the femurs are at an angle of 80° to each other and the legs are bent up at 100° or more (see also table on page 43). In medicine it is usual to give the spread position as half the angle. This means that in medical literature you will find the angle given as 40°, not 80°.

Now for the interesting values during the hip carry. **When babies sit on their mother's hips without a sling, wrap or other carrier, simply supported by an arm around their back, the spread position of the thighs is, on average, 45°! At**

Abduction and adduction angles – conventional information in medicine

With regard to the spread–squat position in medicine:

- the spread angle of the thighs is called the *abduction angle*. This gives the half angle between the two spread thighs, with the value being 0° when the thighs are pressed together. The further the legs are spread, the larger the value.
- the squat, or tuck, angle is called the *adduction angle*. A value of 0° means a stretched leg and the greater the bend of the leg, the greater the angle.

the same time, the legs are often at a right angle, often even more tucked up, particularly in younger babies. The measured spread angle fluctuated in the investigations between a minimum of 36° and a maximum of 56°, with the higher values measured for older babies. The preferred spread angle was, however, 45° (see table on page 43).

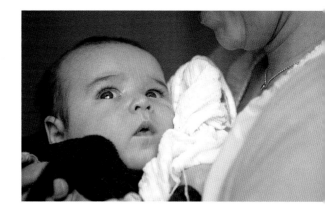

The range of values results from the extent to which the mother carried her children to the side on her hip (which gave lower values) or carried them further forward (which gave higher values, as in the case of the highest measurement of 56°). The legs are bent preferably at 90° to 110°, up to a maximum of 120°. The older children bent their legs less while the higher values were recorded for very young ones.[14]

The comparison of the leg position (with Büschelberger's measurements) that an infant adopts spontaneously during the normal hip carry confirms that the anatomy of the hip joints in infancy is adapted to being carried. During the hip carry, a baby adopts the position in which the femoral head is ideally oriented to the hip-joint socket and fits best to its shape.

An infant carried on the hip spontaneously adopts the ideal leg position for the development of the hip joint. While the thigh is bent at least to a right angle, often even more, the spread angle is an average of 45°. This is a position that promotes the healthy development of the cartilaginous hip joint structures in many ways.

Hip dysplasia and carrying

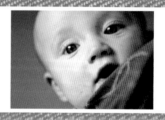

Basic facts about dysplasia

The subject of hip dysplasia and its treatment in children deserves careful consideration. This is because it is one of the most common orthopaedic conditions in infants, although the frequency of occurrence varies significantly between studies. In the case of newborns, it is given as 0.57–3 per cent, as 2–4 per cent or even 1–5 per cent.[15] In addition, the treatment of pronounced dysplasia, which requires the use of hip-abduction pants or other devices commonly used in medicine (if necessary, even a plaster cast on the legs), is a strain for both child and parent. It is not just the fact that the little one must miss out on the unrestricted independent motor activities appropriate to his age. As a result of the medical devices, a baby 'mutates' into a heavy, bulky package. Depending on the situation, in addition to the motor restrictions, the baby may also be deprived

of most of the physical affection from his parents. Depending on the treatment method, it can be difficult to quickly take this awkward bundle into your arms, carry it around or sit it on your lap. Often unconsciously, parents tend to lift up their child less and less as it is such a strain.

Of course, motor development is not restricted to a particular period or to the first year of life. And in the most diverse of areas, it is surprising how well children can recover when they are deprived of experiences in the usual stages of development. However, we should not take strains of this type lightly and should continue to search for alternative treatments that better suit the child.

Even if this condition occurs frequently in some families, a genetic disposition does not play the only role. Even with identical twins, only in 43 per cent of cases did both siblings have a dislocation: in 57 per cent of the cases, they *did not*. As the genetic make-up of identical twins is the same, both siblings would present with the condition if it was purely genetic in origin.[16] Thus hip dysplasia is a concern for any family, as the way and manner in which an infant is handled has a significant influence on whether or not any disposition actually leads to the occurrence of the condition. At this point I don't want to go into the discussion of whether a genetic predisposition is actually necessary, or whether dysplasia or dislocation can be caused by external intervention alone. **If a primarily stretched leg position is forced in the hip joints, an inherited hip-joint socket can be mechanically damaged.** This is because, at this age, stretching the legs causes an awkward orientation of the femoral head to the joint socket and unnatural pressure is exerted on individual areas in the socket. Strains of this type may cause the cartilaginous structures of the

hip joint socket to develop abnormally. The above-mentioned old method of bandaging frequently led to catastrophic hip dislocations caused by the associated stretching in the hip joint area.

Hip dislocations are fortunately very rare in the central European area today as, thanks to awareness from the medical side and the possibility of ultrasound tests, the initial stages of hip dysplasia can be recognised very early. To support the healthy maturation of the hip joint damaged during development, we are mostly restricted to the use of various bandages, adduction pants and so on, which force a slightly spread and tucked up position. The movement of the legs is generally not fully restricted. However, depending on the symptoms, in some cases the legs are fixed in a suitable position using a plaster cast. With therapeutic treatments of this type, a spread–squat position (also known in this context as a 'sit–tuck' position)

	SPREAD POSITION/ ABDUCTION ANGLE	SQUAT POSITION/ ADDUCTION ANGLE
In hip carry position	average of 45°	90° to 120°
Measurements taken with anatomical specimens of newborns – (Büschelberger)[17]	40°	larger than 100°
Medical Guidelines for Hip Dysplasia[18]	30° to 45°	90° to 110°

Table 2 Comparing the values of the spread–squat position.

Congenital hip dysplasia in infancy

The terms congenital dislocation or congenital dysplasia of the hip (CDH), or developmental dysplasia of the hips (DDH), are also used.

At one time the term congenital dysplasia referred to the malposition of the hip joint section in an infant in which an underdeveloped hip joint socket is too shallow and, sometimes, too steep. Nowadays, the term dysplasia also refers to developmental delays or defects and/or to a generally immature hip socket. As the hip joints of an infant are initially cartilaginous structures that are gradually replaced by bone between the third and ninth months of life, dysplasia can also develop from delayed or interrupted ossification. If, in addition, malformed cartilage structures remain undiscovered and also untreated, they ossify in their malformation. Although the frequently used prefix 'congenital' suggests otherwise, dysplasia can also occur a long time after birth.

If dysplasia remains untreated, the hip socket may become even flatter, or shallow, due to the constant adverse pressure of the femoral head on the cartilaginous structures. The discomfort, which will probably only appear in adulthood, may make an operation necessary. In the worst cases of hip dislocation, the femoral head slips out of the joint. Normal walking is then no longer possible as the joint cannot fulfil its function.

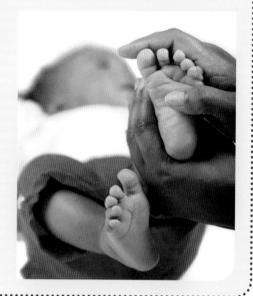

with a spread angle of 30° to 45° is recommended, while the bend should be at least 90° (or even better 100° or even 120°).[19] Do you remember the facts about a baby being carried? **The position recommended by the medical establishment with regard to dysplasia corresponds to the position of the thighs when a baby sits on the hip of an adult!** The spread angle is, on average, 45°, the thighs are usually bent at a right angle, often more so, up to around 120°, particularly with very young infants. Although I repeat myself, I want to stress: during the hip carry, your baby adopts a leg position that corresponds to his anatomical development – and in doing this, also meets the therapeutic requirements for hip dysplasia in a voluntary manner that suits the child's requirements.

Congenital hip dysplasia is one of the most common orthopaedic conditions in infancy. The medical treatment of the condition requires the legs to be adjusted to exactly the same position as the leg position of a baby when carried on the hip. Thus, hip carrying is a suitable way of preventing hip dysplasia in children.

From good and bad traditions – a brief comparison of cultures

The claim that the femoral head is in the ideal position in relation to the hip joint socket when the child is being carried is backed up by investigations that compared various cultures. These found a noticeable link between the occurrence of hip dysplasia or dislocations and the type of childcare.[20] In populations in which infants primarily have or had a stretched leg position due to their type of care, and who were also given less opportunity to move freely, dysplasia or dislocations occurred more frequently. Some North American

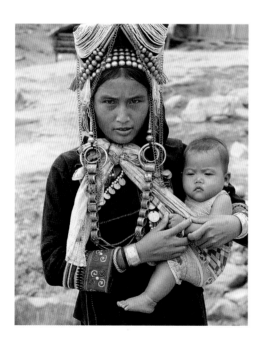

Indian tribes traditionally tie their babies to 'cradleboards'. In Canadian tribes in which this was still common in 1964, 12.3 per cent of babies suffered from dysplasia. In tribes in which their infants were no longer tied to the cradleboards in the traditional manner, the value was just 1.2 per cent at this time – 10 per cent lower![21] **In contrast, in many other cultures in the Asian and African regions, the children were – and still are today – carried with their legs in a tucked and moderately spread position.** They also had more opportunity to move freely.[22] Malformations of the hip joint were almost unknown in these areas.

Just as striking as the comparison of these figures are the observations made by the Japanese doctor Shigeo Nagura. Back in 1940 he pointed out the link between care practices and dysplasia.[23] Due to the traditional methods in which children were often carried with their legs spread and in a tucked position, almost no dislocations were diagnosed in Japan at the start of the last century. But as traditional methods of caring for infants were gradually altered to reflect European conventions, diseases of this type became more and more frequent. As a result of his observations, initially Nagura did not treat children with dislocated hips – as was standard in Europe at this time – with hospitalization and an operation in which the femoral head was reinserted into the socket. Instead, he instructed the parents to carry their children, some of whom were already six months of age, in the traditional Japanese style. Then he documented the development of the hip joints using monthly X-rays – something which would today make the hair of parents and paediatricians stand on end! At that time, however, this was a standard procedure. Nevertheless, he successfully treated the children for dislocated hips without the need for a serious operation. Even though there is no precise data on the seriousness of the hip joint conditions in these case examples, Nagura's achievements show the preventative effect of carrying as well as the therapeutic effect on developed dysplasia. Today, however, Japan has one of the highest rates of hip dysplasia in the world.[24]

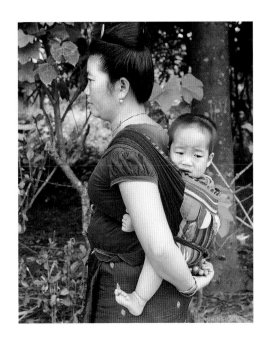

The comparison of cultures in which babies are traditionally carried with their legs tucked up and cultures in which babies spend most of their first year with a stretched body and leg position clearly shows that carrying in the spread–squat position has both a prophylactic and a therapeutic effect on hip dysplasia.

Carrying – a plea for preventative measures against hip dysplasia

As the results of the investigations show, carrying is both a preventative measure and also, in some cases, a child-friendly treatment alternative for hip dysplasia. This is increasingly accepted by physicians – with good reason, if the current definition of the symptoms of dysplasia and the development of the hip joints in childhood is broken down in more detail. **The cartilaginous structures of the hip joint socket and the femoral head are gradually re-placed by bone. They 'mature' continuously between the third and ninth month.** Therefore the correct position of the femoral head in relation to the hip socket during this time is essential for healthy development. Parents should consider that immature hip sockets are described as dysplastic even though they may be simply slow to mature. In other words, the definition may include the delayed ossification of the normal cartilaginous hip socket. In the case of the diagnosis of dysplasia '… the majority of children actually do not require any treatment…',[25] stated the renowned German orthopaedist Ewald Fettweis, as the hip joints actually develop quite normally on their own in most children. This sounds reassuring. The crux of the matter is – and here I defend the doctors – that one cannot know in advance which hip joints will continue to develop normally without any treatment. So as a precautionary measure, children who don't actually need treatment are also treated.[26]

The spontaneous recovery rate – that is, recovery without therapeutic support – is relatively high, depending on the child's age at diagnosis. The percentage is given as 60 or even 80 per cent.[27] This assumes, however, that care practices do not encourage dysplasia. Given these circumstances, adduction pants, Frejka pillows, Pavlik harnesses and the like are still used to treat the condition aggressively today, even though the behaviour of infants, as reported by their parents, is badly affected. In borderline cases in particular, parents assuredly accept carrying their babies as a child-friendly alternative to adduction pants, and the positive effect of carrying is explained to them. Even if the little ones can escape from their physically restrictive devices for a few hours a day, this is still important for their development as, at this age, they also need the essential physical contact and motor stimulation that are restricted to a greater or lesser extent, depending on the treatment method. So sometimes parents are dismissed with the words: 'Your child will pay for your decision later with their

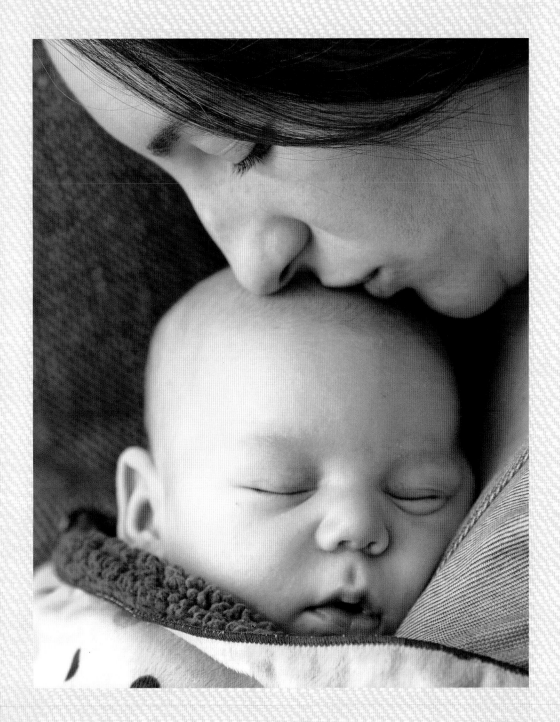

health', when they suggest carrying the baby in the spread-squat position. Only a few parents have the courage to look for alternatives, even though I know some who have courageously and successfully decided to carry their child as a temporary or even only treatment method. I can only recommend asking several doctors for advice to ensure that you consider a wide range of options.

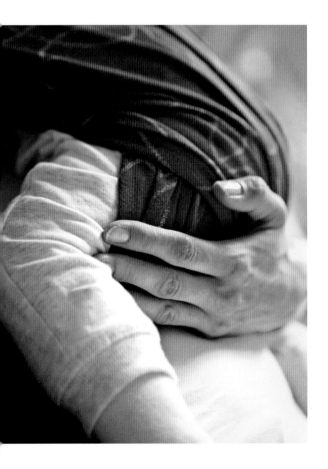

At this point I would particularly like to emphasise that, when carrying the infant on the hip, his hip joints are not *only* held in the optimum position. **Each step taken by the carrying person – particularly when in the lateral hip carry – and each twist and turn of the child, also causes subtle movements in the hip joints of the child.** This encourages healthy development as the cartilaginous structures of the hip joint are better supplied with blood during movement than when in a fixed position. In addition, provided that the femoral head is correctly positioned in relation to the hip socket, movements and the resulting strength and functional strain support the ossification of the entire hip joint system. Although the hip carry in the case of dysplasia is particularly favourable, infants also adopt the ideal leg position when carried to the front, as shown with various measurements taken when using a sling or a wrap.[28] This assumes that the wrap is tied correctly. The legs are so tightly tucked up that the backs of the knees are higher than the nappy. Nowadays, it is always emphasised that the pronounced squat position is more important for the healthy development of the joint structures than the spread position. Particular attention should be paid to the correct squat position.[29]

Paediatricians often instruct parents to use 'broad swaddling' or 'broad diapering', in other words putting on broadly folded broadly folded nappies on their baby if there are signs of dysplasia and to come back for a check-up after a short time. This would be an indication that carrying has a pronounced positive effect, which is altogether fitting. If parents are sure that carrying is a child-friendly – and also parent-friendly – form of care, in which the femoral head is ideally adjusted to the hip socket, some would also be prepared to carry their babies just as a preventative measure. Finally, nowadays, we know that if a family has a predisposition to dysplasia, this represents an increased risk for any baby in the family. Girls are six times more likely to have the condition than boys and it is now one of the most common paediatric orthopaedic conditions. All of this will lead parents to adopt this 'alternative care method' as a precautionary measure, as well, to assure themselves of their 'scrupulousness' in every regard. In the next chapter I will respond to general reservations and fears relating to carrying infants (more on this on page 52).

The spontaneous recovery rate for congenital hip dysplasia is relatively high. Carrying an infant in the spread–squat position provides more than just the ideal orientation of the femoral head to the hip socket. In the hip carry in particular, the still cartilaginous structures are subject to subtle motor stimuli with every step of the parent and each movement of the child, which encourages blood to flow through this area and thus promotes healthy development.

All about babywearing: myths and facts

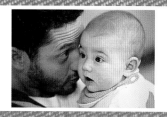

The myth of spinal damage

For many years, babywearing was rarely given any consideration in the European region, despite the research done by Nagura and Büschelberger and culture-comparing observations, and despite the fact that renowned orthopaedists recommended it as a prophylactic measure.[30] Upright carrying was generally only accepted when a baby could sit independently, thus at six months of age at the earliest; otherwise, the spine would be under too much pressure and would be damaged. However, therapeutic measures against dysplasia must be taken as early as possible, often at just a few weeks of age. This time-based discrepancy between acceptance and therapeutic necessity was probably the most important reason for the lack of response to the findings described.

Paediatricians, orthopaedists and physiotherapists feared that early carrying of infants in an upright body position would place too much strain on the spine and cause scoliosis, kyphosis or further posture conditions.[31] Grandparents and other relations were of the same opinion – and sometimes still are today – and thus they demonised this 'new-fangled rubbish'. If carrying is to be accepted as a prophylactic measure in the case of hip dysplasia or in general as an appropriate care method, this objection must be taken seriously and refuted. The extent to which a baby's back could possibly be damaged is still one of the first questions asked by a parent today when they are thinking about babywearing – often in connection with the age from which their little one can be carried upright.

To clarify this at the start: **there is no connection between carrying babies in an upright position and an increase in the frequency of bad posture, posture conditions or spinal damage.** The carrying habits of over 600 parents were recorded in a long-term carrying study.[32] For almost half of the children, information was available up until school age. The questionnaires showed that in the 1980s and 1990s, some mothers initially laid their very young children in the sling or wrap having heard many warning voices. However, two-thirds of the parents switched to the upright carrying method within the first six weeks or used the upright method from the start. In total, half of the children sat in a sling, wrap or other carrier for between one and two and a half hours each day, often even more, during the first four weeks of life. Some were even carried for six hours or more each day. Even when these children were carried upright on a walk or shopping trip during their first week of life, they had no higher occurrence of posture conditions in the spinal area by the time they started school than those who weren't carried.[33] This confirms a medical study carried out recently by the University Clinic, Cologne. In this study, children of school starting age were examined specifically for spinal conditions and the data from 79 children who were carried only rarely or not at all (less than once per week) was compared with that of children who were carried more frequently (41 each day and 59 several times per week).[34]

As the survey of the parents showed, most babies in the long-term study were carried in slings, wraps or other carriers when on walks or when shopping for around two to two and a half hours each day during the first six months of life. There's no fear of later posture conditions or damage occurring. Even with children who were carried sitting and upright for

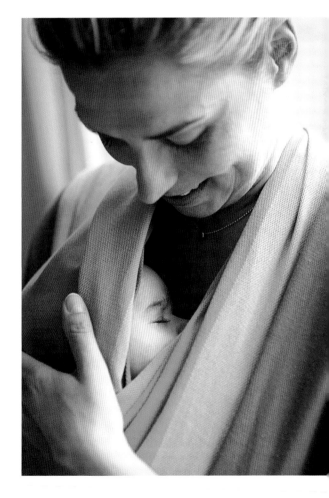

between four and six hours, sometimes even 10 hours, per day as babies (approx. 40 examples), spinal or posture conditions did not occur any more frequently than in children who were not carried. One family in this group is particularly interesting. With one of the children, who was carried for an average of six hours per day as a baby, slight scoliosis was found later – a 'family illness' on the mother's side, which was not considered by the doctor to require treatment. It also occurred with the sibling who was not carried. There was no occurrence with a further sibling who was also carried in the sling or wrap for six hours each day. In this particular family, long-term carrying had, in principle, no negative influence on the development of the back and the spine.[35]

Even with children who spent more than four hours a day (sometimes even six to ten hours) upright in a sling or a wrap, spinal conditions were not found to occur any more frequently at school starting age than the average for the age group in total.

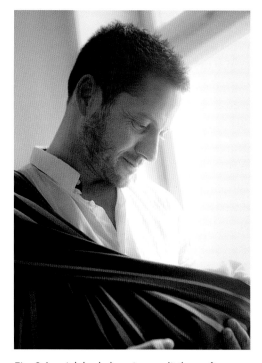

Fig. 8 A quick look: how is your little one?

Facts and fiction – the supply of oxygen to the child

One question that is asked almost as frequently as the one about spine damage is: 'Can the baby get enough air?' Some commentators even claim that children in slings or wraps or other carriers are quiet because they aren't getting enough air and are drowsy because of a lack of oxygen. The question of whether healthy babies would sit peacefully if deprived of air, and actively snuggle their faces into the pullover of mummy or daddy, is one that you can probably only answer yourself. Many mothers turn their baby's head to the side to give him fresh air. However, babies often turn their faces back again of their own accord and press their noses back into the soft pullover that smells of mummy or daddy. In addition, the paediatrician Waltraud Stening and her colleagues at the University Clinic, Cologne[36] showed that the supply of oxygen both to healthy premature babies and full-term babies did not, by any means, reach clinically critical values when the baby was carried upright in a wrap. Only with premature babies did the oxygen saturation of the blood fall slightly – by 0.8 per cent during carrying, compared to the measurements when lying in a pushchair (96.3 per cent compared to 97.1 per cent). **All the same, the oxygen supply to a healthy baby who is being carried upright does not normally vary from that when he is lying down in a pushchair.** I am talking about healthy children and stable premature babies here. I am not referring to 'kangaroo care' for premature babies who can only leave the incubator for a short time and who must remain under intensive medical supervision. I will look at this subject later (see page 90). Nonetheless, investigations of premature babies who are laid upright on the mother or father's breast prove time after time that carrying has a stabilising effect on the breathing and circulatory system.[37]

> With healthy full-term babies, the supply of oxygen during carrying is the same as when lying in a pushchair.

A tiresome question: is the human infant an altricial or clinging young?

Until the 1960s, as already mentioned, a baby was considered to be a passive, helpless being, an 'incomplete construction',[38] more or less only able to eat, sleep, cry and grow. **The abilities of the infant were measured against those of adults or compared with the characteristics of the offspring of related animal species.** Compared directly with the young of the great apes most closely related to us, such as chimpanzees, bonobos or gorillas, a human baby comes off quite badly overall and appears decidedly helpless. In the 1960s and 1970s, comparative morphology and anthropology highlighted the fact that an infant in its first year of life is not capable of anything considered typical for a human in terms of posture, movement or communication abilities.[39] Of course, compared to the abilities of an adult, deficiencies are bound to be apparent. The physical characteristics of human offspring appear to be more reminiscent of an altricial species, in other words young dogs or cats – parents should forgive these researchers – than the young of the closest related species to us, the great apes, who can hold onto their mothers or crawl around them. Therefore, initially the human infant was classified as an example of altricial young. However, this was by no means satisfactory, as after all, altricial species are born more immature in more ways than just their ability to move. Their behaviour, even at the age at which they can already explore their environment, offers significant contradictions (see page 22).

Comparative observations – particularly of great apes – also breathed life into the scientific assessment of human babies. Ape and great ape offspring were in fact affiliated with the precocial group. This is the young type which, as a newborn, tries to follow the mother on wobbly legs just a few minutes after birth like, for example, foals or elephant calves. This requires coordinated movement, fully functioning sensory organs and a generally mature state of development. Even though they cannot run after the adult animals, ape off-spring are assigned to this group due to their comparable physiological maturity and because they actively hold onto their mother. They also showed the characteristics described at the start (see also page 22) during their prenatal development: the growing foetus passes through a sort of 'altricial stage' in the uterus.

As a result of the close relationship and this characteristic during the prenatal time, the 'human young' also had to be counted as one of the precocial group. However, as before, its helplessness was irritating in comparison to the chimpanzee young, for

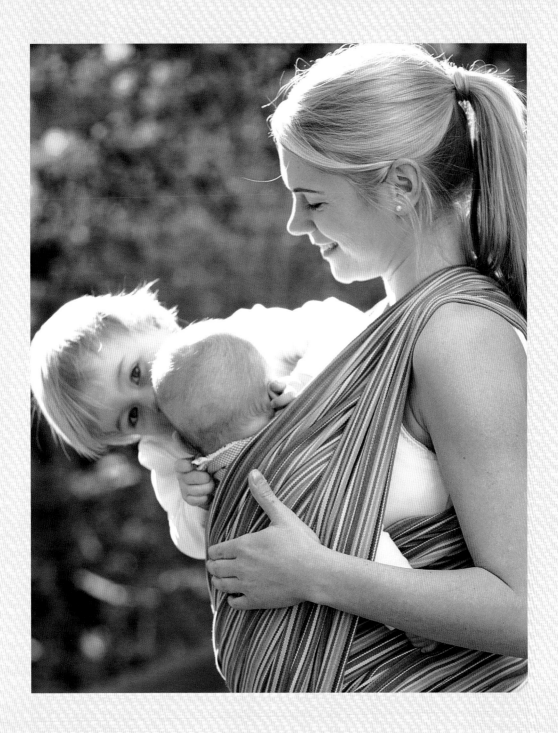

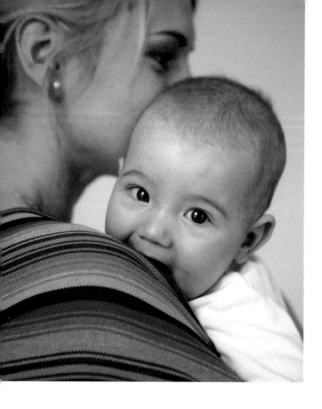

all the investigations and discussions, there it was: the assessment of helpless altricial young.

With the observation that 'a baby is a secondary altricial type', the scientific discussion was luckily not yet closed. So why don't I just start with the year 1970, when the Freiburg biologist Bernhard Hassenstein defined the third young type of 'clinging young' and assigned the human infant to this group?[41] The reason is the persistence with which the most diverse of disciplines still consider that a child is best suited to the lying position. Even today I receive emails in which it is claimed that nurses or physiotherapists only permit the lying position for carrying in the first three months of life. The suitability of carrying human babies is thus being fundamentally disputed, but with no scientific basis. **Due to the characteristic linked features and behaviour, the fatal classification of the human infant to the altricial group thus bypasses the basic needs of a child.** Altricial young are left alone in their nest by their mothers for hours on end and they are suited to this. The high fat content of the milk of the altricial mother guarantees that the young are full for a correspondingly long time. The fat content of the milk of the mothers of clinging young, and thus of humans, is much lower in comparison, as the offspring originally had constant access

example. The immature appearance at birth, the inability to communicate or to move 'as per the species' ultimately caused the Basel biologist Adolf Portmann to assign the human infant a special status within its relationship.[40] Thus, originally 'intended' as a precocial species, the time of birth of the offspring in the course of the specific evolution of humans was brought forward and thus, in comparison to the original planned birth state, it was ever more immature when born. As an 'intended' premature birth with regard to evolutionary history, he thus is effectively born as an altricial species, even if secondary. So after

to the source of food. At least, this was what biology intended. Here one could discuss breastfeeding and feeding on demand, but I would like to restrict myself to referring to the relevant literature.[42] One reference should, however, be mentioned at this point. An initial investigation appeared to indicate that carrying influenced the breastfeeding behaviour of the mother. Babywearing mothers breastfeed more frequently and for longer overall.[43]

The comparison of behaviour in alarming situations also shows the discrepancy between these two types of young. As soon as young wolves or foxes are agile enough to explore the environment, they return to the protective burrow if there is danger and do not search for their mother. This is in complete contrast to little Goma, the famous gorilla in Basle (see page 22), or all other ape young. If they are distressed, they look for the closeness and safety of their mother. And the same applies for little *Australopithecus* and humans.

To describe a human baby as altricial is scientifically outdated and neglects the basic biological needs and behavioural characteristics of a baby, which in all its behavioural facets and other characteristics belongs within the type of clinging young.

Child-friendly, natural 'early-learning support'

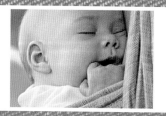

Babywearing: perception of parents with the senses

Why does babywearing have such a calming effect?[44] Because almost all senses are activated during carrying. Specifically, your baby senses your movements and your physical proximity directly: these are the most intensive signals that confirm your presence to him. He hears – and feels – your voice and the sound of you breathing. The heartbeat is a rhythm that is familiar from the prenatal period. In addition, your facial features are in the optimum range of vision when he is being carried[45] – about 20 to 25cm (8 to 10 in) away from him. As a result, your baby can observe your facial expressions and thus get to know you and your reactions in different situations. In the same way, your smell becomes familiar to him. We generally underestimate sensory perception as it often has a subconscious influence. Even on the second day of life, newborns preferred the smell of their own mother over other breastfeeding mothers, provided that they were able to get to know them sufficiently through frequent and close physical contact.[46] In our society this learning efficiency can be obstructed by our usual clothing, yet after a few days infants still recognise the specific smell of their mother even if, for example, it is overpowered by perfume. The little ones learn particularly well when they have direct skin contact with the people they trust.[47]

When babywearing, you offer your child a whole range of sensory stimuli, and your baby can soon link the individual components to you on a personal level. Furthermore, the stimulation of the different senses is more than just 'perception at the respective sensory level', this applies, in particular, to the tactile senses, thus the perception of touch, and the sensory system, which is responsible for movement and self-perception, the so-called proprio-vestibular sense. Both sensory systems deserve more consideration so that we can fully appreciate and take into account their significance for a child's development.

Almost all of a baby's senses are stimulated during carrying. Tactile and proprio–vestibular stimulation is not only a good calming mechanism, it is also particularly important during the development of the child and his abilities.

The proprio-vestibular sensory system – a little-known but all-pervading wonder

Vestibular and proprioceptive perception gives information about the position of one's own body in a space, about the position and changes to position of the individual body parts in relation to each other and about their movement and direction of movement. The proprio-vestibular system encompasses the sense of balance, location and movement whereby information about the activity of participating muscles and tendons is also included.

Proprioceptive perception is used as a synonym for deep sensibility, kinaesthetic sensibility and self-perception. The vestibular system, also known as the sense of balance, is closely related to the processing centres of the neck and eye muscles.

Skin contact – food for body and soul

When you breastfeed, embrace, stroke and caress your baby, you are sending particularly intense messages about your attentiveness and devotion. Tactile sensory perception is one of the most important channels of communication for a baby and is essential for normal development. There have been a number of investigations into the effects of adequate tactile perception on the overall development of a child – some almost bordering on miraculous. In this regard, premature babies in particular were investigated. Repeated short massages, for example, for three-quarters of an hour each day over the course of two weeks, were enough to help low-weight premature babies gain almost twice as much weight than those who received no massages, even though the quantity of food given was the same.[48] The premature babies who had the pleasure of this skin stimulation were awake and active for a longer time – much to the surprise of the observers, who had initially claimed that the increase in weight was due to longer, calmer periods of sleep. The intensive contact was, in fact, the reason why the intake of food was easier, and additionally the food could be better utilised. Investigations of the physiology of metabolism have confirmed this effect,

which was initially rather puzzling. Intensive tactile sensory perception causes the distribution of various endogenous substances and these, in turn, permit the improved utilisation and application of the food. In addition, tactile stimulation means less susceptibility to stress, so overall babies are calmer and more balanced.[49] **Such intensive tactile perceptions are 'food for the soul', which can be interpreted as grams/ounces in body weight.**

Although premature babies probably benefit more from such 'calming units' due to their special situation – after all, their needs are significantly greater – the benefits also apply to healthy infants. Thus some authors treat massage as not only a traditional remedy for flatulence and similar problems, they also describe the positive effect on breathing, the circulatory system and temperature regulation. Like premature babies, normal-weight babies who are regularly massaged are more responsive, attentive and capable after just a few weeks. They feel comfortable in their environment more quickly, are more sociable and easier to settle in various ways and their motor skills are generally more developed.[50] What is also striking here is their high level of self-regulation. All these factors simplify the handling of a baby, facilitate interaction between parent and child and thus support the overall development of the baby, as well as the emotional relationship between the team of two or three. And incidentally, this close physical contact with the baby also influences the parent. **As skin-to-skin contact with the baby helps to produce stress-reducing hormones, it also calms the mother.**[51]

Although 'professional' massages were the focus – scientific evidence requires standardised conditions and thus a precise number of 'physical contact units' – normal pleasurable, emotional cuddles with an infant should by no means give way to such fixed massage patterns. 'Excessive snuggling after a bath, 'cuddle attacks' on the changing mat – your baby enjoys this physical closeness and the resulting affection. He needs the focused emotional devotion and attention to be able to feel, bit by bit, absolutely sure of the emotional attachment. This form of contact helps the baby to develop a body schema or a model of the body just as much as the massages. **Children who are allowed to experience their body in a positive way can also build a positive self-image.** Thus youths and adults who experience physical devotion in an exuberant and positive way, in this way affirming their body, feel more attractive, body aware and more receptive to physical touch. This carries particular weight during puberty and in subsequent

relationships with a partner. These findings were included in sex education books as well as in therapies for physically abused children and in treatment of children with depressive mothers who, at least for a time, kept their distance from the child.[52]

Against the background of this almost unbelievable list of positive effects of massage and skin contact, we should remind ourselves what a baby would be

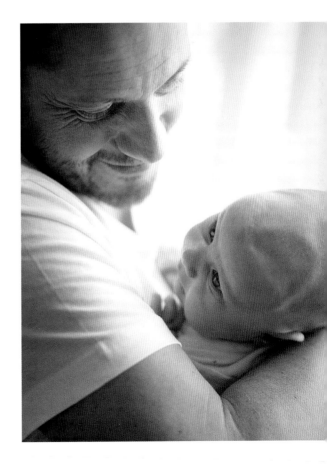

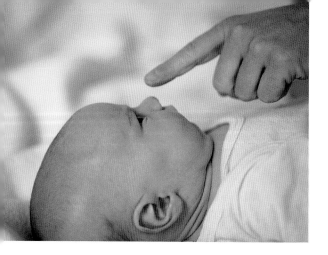

deprived of with the traditional, but still common, methods of baby care if he reacts in such a strong and measurable way to such physical contact. **To sleep alone in his bed, to see the world from a pushchair at a greater physical distance from his attachment figure, to initially vaguely perceive the parents at the other end of this vehicle, does not in any way meet the natural needs of a baby.** If this represents the 'main offer' for a child in the first months of life, interrupted by comparatively short periods of physical contact when a nappy is changed, for example, and without frequent breastfeeds, it is no surprise that we hear vehement signs of dissatisfaction from a baby lying in a pushchair or a bouncy chair.

Intensive, frequent skin and physical contact supports the physical development of a baby in the most diverse of ways. The children are also more sociable, they cry less, can cope better with stressful situations and also have a better ability to self-regulate.

Unnoticed but fundamental: the sense of movement and balance

Being moved means stimulation of the proprio-vestibular system. This is the sense of balance and speed as well as self-perception of the body (see page 61). As adults we are often unaware of the significance of this uninterrupted active perception – unless we are tripping over our own feet because we have had one glass of sparkling wine too many, while drinking to the health of a new addition to the human race! Although, in the truest sense of the word, this system accompanies us at every turn, the phenomena of smell, taste, hearing, seeing and touching – the classical senses – are usually more familiar. However, in the development of a child, the proprio-vestibular system has particular significance, as research in recent decades has proven. The balance organs develop in the sixth to eighth weeks of pregnancy. In addition to the tactile system, the proprio-vestibular sensory system is also one of the first functioning senses in the development of a human. As early as the fourth week of development, an embryo can react to contact stimuli, and foetal movements can be seen at just six weeks. At twelve weeks, the pattern of movements, which was initially puppet-like, changes. Reactions become more fluid even though the relevant parts of the brain only take control in the middle of the pregnancy. A foetus can therefore sense early tactile stimulations, as well as situation and position changes of his own body, as well as his mother's. However, for the subsequent development of the sensory system, he also needs the appropriate stimuli over and over again.[53]

Being jiggled around moves the little world of a newborn just like physical contact in the familiar world of the uterus. This is why, since time immemorial, parents have used cradles to rock their children to sleep. However these practical 'devices' had a bad reputation for many years and they were banned from children's rooms under the guise of spoiling the child. Since the 1980s, however, they have

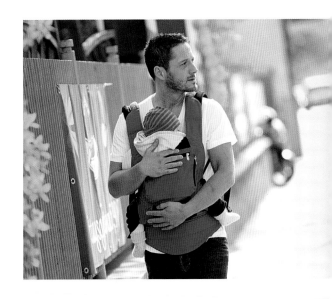

gradually recaptured their ancestral ground in the form of traditional cradles, special baby hammocks, hanging cradles and other similar products. Cradles simulate being carried by a caring person. To investigate the phenomenon of these treasured pieces of furniture, or rather the calming effect of 'movement', scientists initially looked at single factors. It would be rather long-winded to list all of these individual results. Ultimately, thanks to these observations, special hammocks and waterbeds found their way into clinics to support the development of newborns and premature babies.[54]

The distinction between movement and physical contact in various investigations is initially confusing. However, this preparatory work was necessary to move away from isolated ways of looking at things and towards an understanding of the interaction of senses. It was ultimately proven that the combination of different stimuli was more effective than individual sensations – and not only in calming an infant but also in terms of their physical development. In neonatal wards, the introduction of waterbeds was followed by the playback of sounds like a heartbeat rhythm and correspondingly rhythmic music.[55]

The realisation that the ideal combination of sensory stimulation was imparted by the parents themselves or by other related persons ultimately triumphed in more and more clinics. 'Old Anna', whom Ashley Montagu reported on in an anecdote and who was summoned to the children's clinic time after time to hold the babies when medical intervention no longer helped, is just one example. It shows how a baby can quite simply respond to the sensory perceptions and stimuli presented to him by sensitive people.

As a result of stimulation of the proprio-vestibular system, babies are calmer and more balanced. This supports physical development and moves the baby's world closer to its usual envisaged environment, as 'intended' by evolution.

The interaction of the senses: the magic term 'multisensory integration'

To be cuddled, caressed and carried in the arms of his parents gives the baby a flood of stimulating sensory perceptions, but they also need to be processed. **To be able to structure and arrange perceived sensory stimuli and place them in a relationship with each other is necessary so that one can orientate oneself and cope in the world.** The cognitive achievements are summarised under the term 'multisensory integration'. The processing of varied perceptions in the central nervous system – in specific associated areas of the brain – enables an individual to react to the different stimuli in the environment in a controlled and coordinated manner.[56] The brain already functions as a central switch point a long time before birth. Even as early as the third month of development, the tactile and balance senses function. In other words, the associated perception structures (sensory organs) and functional switch units (nerve cells or neurons) are formed and process perceived signals.

However, a sensory system can only function/function better if it is used; otherwise it gradually wastes away. If it is regularly presented with appropriate stimuli, the neurons in the associated region of the brain are stimulated into growth and more and more connections (synapses) are created between the individual nerve cells. The interaction of stimuli and the reactions of the body can thus function in a more developed, complex and perfect manner. An improved network of neuronal connections develops, which reacts more quickly and is more adapted to individual requirements. However, the individual regions of the brain related to sensory perception influence one another. A stimulated sensory system always has an effect on the region of the brain associated with other perception systems. The more that sensory systems are stimulated, the

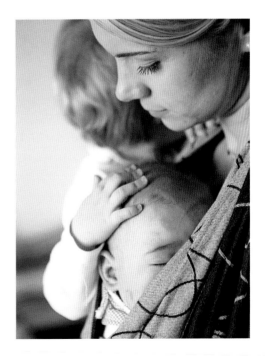

more the individual regions of the brain are further structured and the better the coordination of different senses with each other – and thus the more developed the overall reactions to the stimulus become.

A newborn's brain weighs only one-fifth of that of an adult, yet he is born with almost all the neurons that he will have in the future. However, the network pattern of the neurons in the brain of a newborn does not, in any way, match that of an adult. The connections are only created and channelled in accordance with appropriate use. Birth brings a greater variety of stimuli, through which a child can develop further. Millions of neurons are just waiting to be able to connect to each other.

The brain of a baby requires constant information from its environment so that these billions of connections can be formed and in the correct way. However, the stimuli must be presented correctly and in a time frame that corresponds to the development of the child. There are so-called 'time windows' for the development of different abilities. If these periods of time pass without the required stimuli and information being offered, the windows can close without being used and the corresponding parts of the brain lie idle, sometimes for ever. This has been proven for the optical sense. For example, a child whose eyes, for medical reasons, could only perceive light stimuli after an operation at three years of age, would remain blind, as the necessary neural connections were not created in the associated sensitive phase and the corresponding parts of the brain intended for the processing of visual stimuli did not develop. Normally, however, if the required stimuli are presented outside of the time window intended for the development, they can still be used, although probably with some limitations. Sometimes stimulation at the wrong time can even hinder development, usually if presented too early and too forcefully. If the range of stimuli is presented too late, however, the parts of the brain can be reactivated, with greater or fewer deficits and developed abilities that lag behind what would actually have been possible.

This knowledge about developmental 'windows' should not prompt you to organise a detailed learning programme for your child. **The windows for different abilities vary greatly and usually last for years.** Generally, a protective and positive stimulating family environment provides everything that a child needs for his development, because normally the basic needs of our offspring are taken into account. For example, for motor development, a period of four years is given. However, if a child only got the chance to move adequately at a much later point, he would still be able to walk, although he would probably be less coordinated. There were reports of an Asian 'wolf child' who was apparently abandoned at a very young age and learned to stand upright and walk after several years. However, he moved in an awkward way and when he wanted to move forwards quickly, he fell back into the four-legged gait which was usual for him.[57]

We should always be aware that specific stimuli at the appropriate time and in the appropriate quantity – there can be too little or too much – offer the optimum chance of development for a child. In our urban environment in which physical freedom is very restricted, children do not have enough opportunity to move freely, often for years at a time.[58] We should counteract this early – and we should encourage physical development as early as possible by carrying our young.

The many perceptions that flood the baby must be structured, arranged and connected to each other (i.e. sensory integration) so that the baby can react to the different stimuli in a sensible, controlled and coordinated way. If the sensory systems are adequately stimulated – in other words, age-appropriately and to the required degree – this creates the optimum preconditions for the child's development.

Babywearing – 'special early years education'

This is nothing new and it continues throughout life: **cognitive performance is increased through more demanding physical activities.** Movement, in particular when new and varied challenges must continuously be overcome, generally leads to the formation and growth of nerves. If nerve cells and their interconnections in the brain of an adult respond to physical activities, it is hardly surprising that corresponding stimuli are much more significant for a brain that is in a stage of development and growth. As mentioned, neuronal structures that are rarely or never used revert or do not develop at all. With this background, it is actually only logical that the 'famous' proprio-vestibular system is assigned such importance in the development of the childhood brain. An example for clarification: imagine that you are jumping up and down. The fact that the cupboard in your field of vision is not moving up and down before your eyes and always appears to you to be fixed on the floor should not be taken for granted, although it seems like that to us. Your understanding that the furniture remains where it is is due to your brain knowing both the position of your body in the room and the position of each part of your body. It then places them in relation to each other.

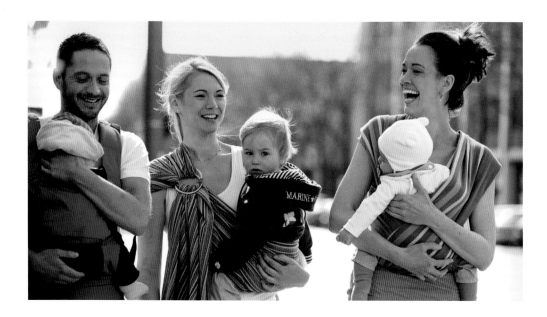

In other words, the head, the body and the leg position, as well as the eye position and movement, are all coordinated with each other. The fact that the proprio-vestibular system is connected to the optical perception area also ensures that we can grab specific things – something that our babies perfect through repeated effort and astonishing concentration.[59] **The links between optical perception, head and eye movements, and hand and arm movements – in other words, complete hand-eye coordination – show how important the proprio-vestibular complex is for the further development of the child in other areas.** And it appears also to 'liven up' the overall development of the brain if stimulated accordingly. For this purpose a test was carried out in which three- to thirteen-month-old babies were spun back-and-forth, ten times in each direction, using a revolving chair. The babies were keen participants in these revolving chair sessions, which only took place four times a week. Although the entire test only lasted four weeks, the differences from the children who did not take part in the revolving action were significant. The 'revolving group' were physically more advanced with sitting, crawling, standing and walking, and also with their reflexes. The results for a pair of twins were particularly interesting. They were four

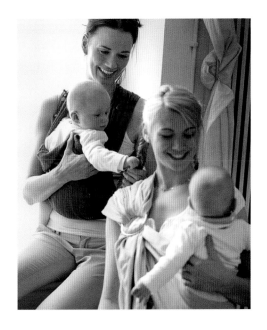

months old when the study ended. The 'trained' twin could already hold his head upright and sit unaided, whereas, in contrast, the 'untrained' twin was just beginning to lift his head.[60]

But back to the subject of carrying. The results of this investigation can be seen as an explanation for the long-standing observation that in various African cultures children carried can stabilise their heads significantly earlier and are more advanced in their motor development than children who have grown up in the West.[61] This is a concrete example demonstrating that a system that is constantly stimulated is also encouraged in its development. Being carried requires more physical activity from a baby and also makes different physical demands than lying in a pushchair. **When a baby is carried, his proprio-vestibular system is not only activated more intensively, but the baby is also presented with more and different stimuli than in a pushchair.** The baby does not simply follow the movements of his parents, which are dependent on different factors, but he must also constantly make many small balancing movements that are necessary just because of the upright body position.

Some scientists argue that the rate of the proprio-vestibular system goes further than enticing the development of the other sensory and motor skills. They consider this sense to be the 'pacemaker' for the interaction of all sensory systems, intrinsic to the complete development of the brain, both at the *neuronal* and *cognitive* levels. As one of the earliest developing sensory systems, it provides a growing being with one of the first sensory experiences of all – during the prenatal period.[62] All subsequent experiences are founded on this early world of experience. Thus they are not only important for sensory and motor skills, because they also influence the subsequent mental development as a cumulative process and also the emotional development, albeit indirectly. Nowadays, as well as knowing about the interactive effects of a damaged sense of balance and delayed motor skills, we also know that perception, learning and concentration problems are also indirectly related. For a long time, various movement and touch therapies have been used to treat behavioural problems and learning difficulties.[63] It doesn't require many intellectual acrobatics to imagine that carrying a baby has just as good an effect – possibly even better – on the child's development. During this time, stimuli such as carrying are almost intended by evolution for the development of the individual.

> The proprio-vestibular and the tactile systems have great importance for a child's development: They are seen as the motor and coordinator for over-coming varied development tasks that can only serve their purpose if they receive constant stimulation.

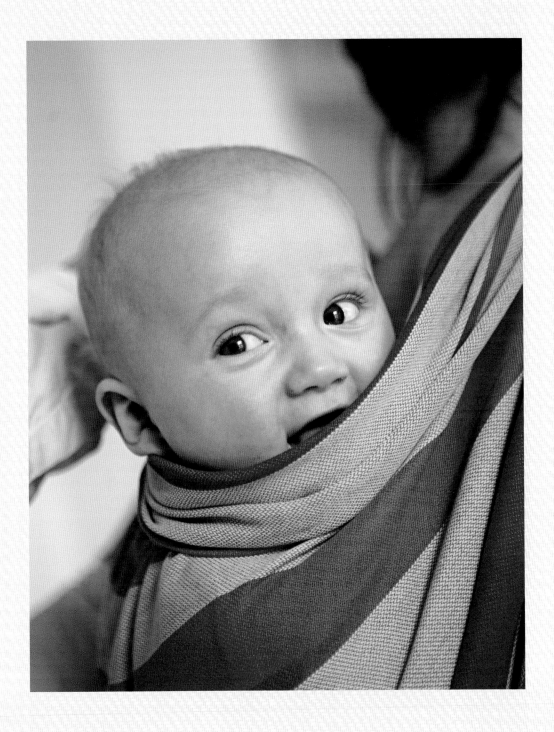

The importance of the parent–child relationship

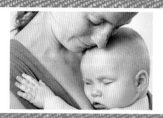

Babywearing – a cornerstone of successful development

Babywearing enriches both the child *and* the parent. On the one hand, the baby, happily snuggled up, receives the 'development programme' that is appropriate to the child and his age. On the other hand,

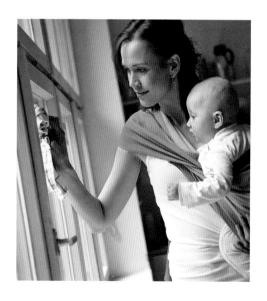

the mother, who is usually initially responsible for everyday care of the child, has, in the truest sense of the words, more of a free hand. The fact that daily stress is reduced is an important argument and cannot be overlooked in everyday family life. **Hectic and overloaded lives, and tension often hinder the development of the emotional relationship between the parent and child.** Excessive demands and stress create a modern-day double-edged sword of Damocles that hangs threateningly over some mother–child teams, as they have such a significant effect on the development of a successful parent–child relationship.[64] Parents need to have at their disposal all conceivable tools to enable them to better master daily life with their child, who they can sometimes find quite exhausting. And they need as much help as possible to reassure them that they are coping well in their role as a parent and to enable them to quickly develop an emotional relationship with this new member of the family. This, in turn, develops the attachment between the child and the parent as the behaviour of the parents initially forms the living environment for the baby. They give him the feeling of security with which he can experience his environment and explore it step by step. A baby learns from the first day of life – and, in particular, learns about all facets of his parents. As well as your appearance and your voice, the baby also registers your behaviour and reactions to his signals. The baby notices whether the parents are available and able to meet his needs in a responsive and appropriate manner. **It is the parents who lay the foundation for the way in which a baby experiences and evaluates his little world, and whether or not he can be sure that his needs are met and he will always receive protection, affection and safety.** They are initially the people who set the framework within which their baby feels more or less embedded and accepted. They give him his own meaning and effectiveness – but also determine whether or not he feels helpless and completely at the mercy of the demands of his environment. As parents, you open up the world of feelings to your baby. Based on his experiences in the first few months of life, a child develops his

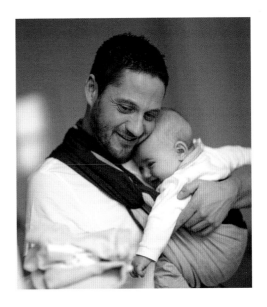

attachment to you and to other reliable interaction partners at around six months.

It is undeniable that a successful parent–child relationship is extremely important for the development of any person: after all we belong to a social species. Children who can be sure of the loving care of adults are more balanced, less anxious and less frequently aggressive. In addition, they are socially competent and know how to assess the limits of their room for manoeuvre. They promptly seek help as soon as a challenging situation threatens, and so they can also better overcome difficult situations.[65] It is easier to deal with children like these. It is absolutely in the parents' own interests to ensure that a child has a secure attachment to them.

We should also clarify again that, as well as being important for child development over-all, the development of the parent–child relationship also determines the range of feelings in many areas in adulthood. In frightening situations, children without a secure attachment react in different ways to those who have one. For example, when separated from parents in an unfamiliar environment, firstly they are more distressed and, secondly, their anxiety lasts for significantly longer. Overall, they have a less suitable strategy for coping in stressful situations. If this is the same throughout childhood, it is hardly surprising that such children also find stressful situations harder to cope with as adolescents and adults.[66] It is true that nowadays we no longer talk about the irreversible, all-deciding first year (or years) of life; however, experiences faced during the early stages of childhood have a significant effect on the development of the personality, because each further development is based on the previous stage of life. If the start of the emotional relationship between the parent and child can be formed successfully, the foundations are laid for the child's subsequent successful development.

A successful relationship means that a child can develop a feeling of security and trust. A positive parent–child relationship is initially mostly based on the sensitivity and the responsiveness of the mother and father. They give their child access to the world and to their feelings, but also to his own.

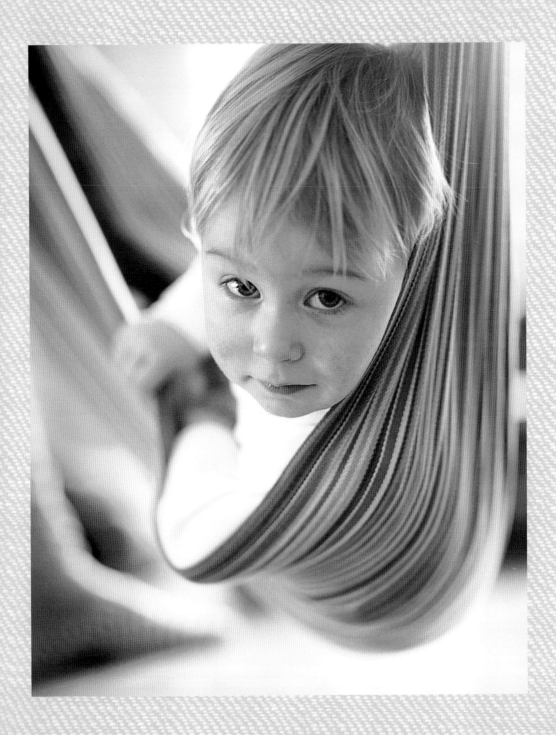

It takes two: the start of the bond and attachment

Nowadays it is indisputable that the hours immediately after birth are a particularly sensitive time for initial contact and the formation of the first emotional ties between mother and child. If intensive physical contact and interaction is possible during this time, the development of the relationship between the mother and her child is facilitated and supported. Mothers can attune themselves more easily to this unknown little person. There are less likely to be breastfeeding problems, in particular

with the first suckling attempts by the newborn. Mothers feel more confident looking after the baby, need less help in everyday situations and want to have their baby with them more often.[67]

However, immediate intense contact after birth is by no means an indispensable precondition for the development of a good parent–child relationship. If a mother has ample opportunity to look after her newborn during the days after his birth, the impact of an initial missed chance can be redressed. Nature deals in second chances. But this does not mean that the opportunity for early contact should be

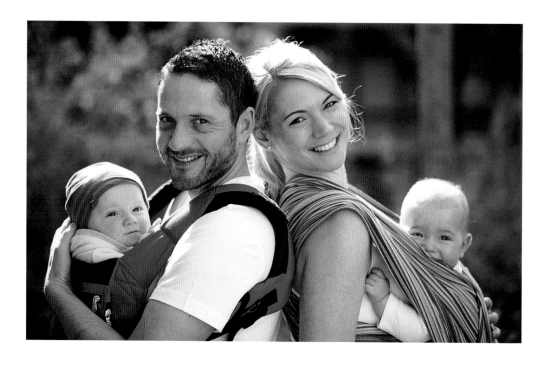

passed up! The smaller participant also plays an important role. He cries a lot more frequently when separated from his mother after the birth. In addition, he also suffers more from all the excitements of his first few days of life: if subjected to stress, his agitation lasts longer and is more intense. The logical consequence of this is that a newborn should stay with his mother whenever possible. If circumstances do not allow this and the father is available immediately after the birth, he can just as successfully take on this initial care role. He is, after all, normally an important and constant relationship partner for a baby. Even if the mother is the focus of interest in all the research, fathers can just as successfully become the initial interaction partner for a newborn.[68] **Neither intuitive parenting nor bonding are the sole domain of the mother.** It is not without reason that scientists have switched from using the term 'mother–child relationship' to using 'parent–child relationship'. I know some fathers to whom this task fell immediately after birth and who took on initial contact with the baby. Even years later, they describe their relationship with this child as much more emotional compared to that with their other children.

A baby is more settled when he stays with his parents after the birth and can enjoy as much physical contact and closeness as possible. And we return to the subject of how can one get to know this little person as quickly and as well as possible when he can't do the one thing that usually makes us understand each other – speak? Using a sling or a wrap instead of a pushchair is a good choice here. Mothers and fathers both benefit as much as their baby if he is in direct proximity as much as possible. When carrying in direct physical contact, the parents feel every stirring and movement of the infant, whether he is sleepy or curious, whether he is unsettled and will soon announce his hunger or whether he will soon fill his nappy. All this is easy to sense when the little one is sitting wrapped up and in close contact. A mother described how she 'still felt a little bit pregnant' when her baby was tied round her so closely.

Such close contact, as often as possible, is the best way of meeting the list of prerequisites for a successful parent–child relationship. The parents have to react to the child's signals in 'a timely and appropriate, reliable and prompt, sensitive and age-appropriate manner'. When, due to this closeness, the mother can sense in advance that her little one is stirring, for example, and will wake soon and that probably the next feed is also due, she can also keep an eye out for a suitable feeding place in good time. A baby can show his needs in more ways than by just grizzling and crying. His range of noises increases quickly, but he also progressively uses body language to communicate. No baby normally turns from a bundle of joy in one instant to a squawking, unpleasant child in the next. Small signals are usually given out before the crying starts, and these can be used as an 'early warning system' if they are noticed. **To be able to react in an anticipatory way makes dealing with an infant less problematic. This has a significant influence on the emotional relationship between the parent and the child.** A settled, generally satisfied child confirms that the mother and father are competent parents and are coping well with their new role. Parents are then less stressed and the baby is also less stressed when he has the occasional bad day.

With their first child, parents in our culture usually have absolutely no experience of dealing with a baby. Everything is new, nights are short, tiredness is constantly an issue, the baby is still a puzzle and his signals are by no means clear at first. The combination of the unknown and uncertainty is not a good basis for coping with the range of tasks required of parents. It also makes it hard to activate the parents' biological resources – intuitive parenting. The spirit is willing but the flesh – or rather the mother – is weak. And yet she is still supposed to react to every signal in a friendly, joyful, prompt, sensitive manner?

Let's get to the point: babywearing helps. Every babywearing mother had this experience before the Elizabeth Anisfeld research group carried out its now classic studies. But it is still reassuring that it is scientifically proven.[69] First it must be highlighted that this research was carried out in families in poor socioeconomic groups, for whom the development of the parent–child relationship could be considered more critical. Mothers were approached in the hospital. One group was shown how to use a soft baby carrier and asked to carry their baby in it regularly in future. The other group received an infant seat, which the mother could use to carry the child around or place next to her. During the first year of life, the behaviour of the mothers and children was observed at regular intervals. At the age of one year, the attachment of the children was classified according to standard tests used in development psychology. In summary, babywearing mothers became more responsive and sensitive to their children and reacted to their needs with more understanding, than the mothers in the control group, although the carrying aids were, on average, used only three times a week. The more positive attitude of the babywearing mothers was also reflected in the attachment behaviour of the one-year-olds in the final investigations. Significantly

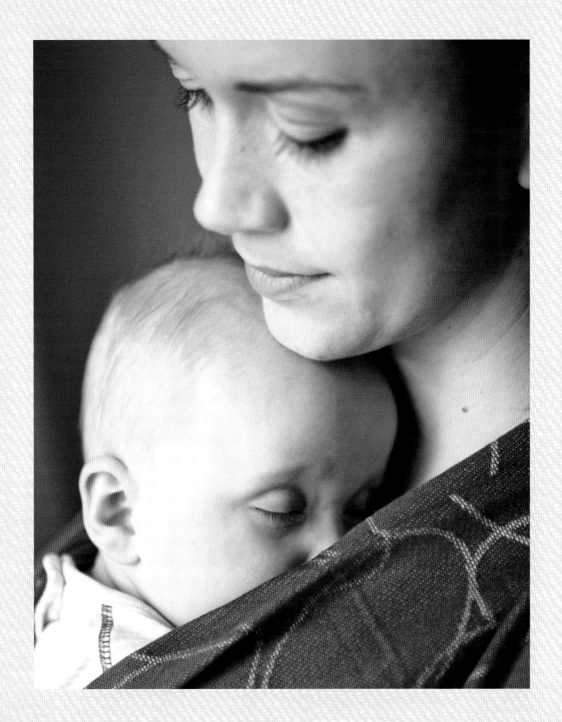

more of the carried children developed a secure attachment to their mothers. Of course, some secure attachment relationships had also formed in the control group, and likewise, there were some poorly attached relationships in the carried group. But the higher rate of secure attachment for the carried children was statistically significant.

Babywearing is not a necessity, and it is also no guarantee of a successful parent–child relationship, but it offers a good opportunity to create a secure relationship. Against this background, the secondary findings of this study are also particularly interesting. After the hospital stay, three mothers in the control group chose to use soft baby carriers of their own accord, which the observers learned about in the course of the study. These three children turned out to be securely attached within the control group.

So parents were affected positively when they had the chance to have their child close by in physical contact. However, this does not only apply to social behaviour. Here is a short example from the large range of studies on premature babies, which gave interesting insights into the significance of physical contact. The American doctor Gene Anderson reported that the mother's temperature initially rose as soon as she laid her premature baby directly onto the skin of her breast, and the body temperature of the baby soon followed suit. As soon as the baby reached a particular temperature, his mother's temperature returned to its normal level. However, it increased again as soon as the child began to cool. When they had their babies close to them, the mothers functioned almost like a thermostat, which kept the child stable at the optimum body temperature.[70] At this point, I would like to

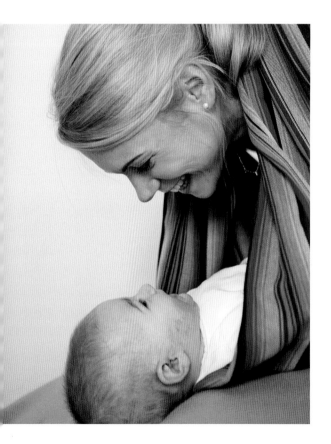

return to the study that links babywearing with the duration and frequency of breastfeeding. Mothers who carried their baby around for just one hour each day breastfed for longer in comparison to mothers who only received breastfeeding advice (at two months: 72 per cent versus 51 per cent; five months: 48 per cent versus 24 per cent). They also breastfed their babies more frequently.[71]

Regular intensive contact between parent and child enables parents to learn about their baby, who is initially rather puzzling, and so encourages the positive development of the attachment and bonding process. Carried children are often more securely attached to their parents. Those who carry their child can develop a more sensitive awareness of the small signals sent by their newborn. In direct physical contact, they can sense the state of their baby and react more sensitively to their child.

Gather experience from outside your own baby's capabilities

Babies and parents are a complementary team. With the support of mum and dad, a child can reach his full potential. Perhaps an example relating to motor development would be helpful here. Infants of only a few days old cannot yet hold their heads up themselves. However, if you hold your baby in an almost upright position (for example if you lay him on your lower arms and hold his head with both hands to support it), he is free from the task of keeping his head under control and stabilising it against the force of gravity. In addition, he shows patterns of movement (albeit supported) that are otherwise normally shown only

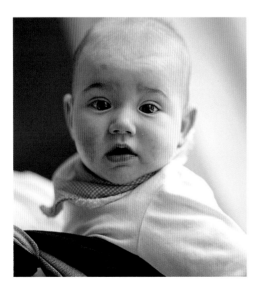

two to three months later.[72] So this upright position stimulates increased attentiveness and increased interest in the environment. Excited by the stimulation of the sense of balance, babies only a few days old willingly follow visual stimuli and also process them better than is usually expected for this age.[73] Parents often subconsciously use this effect to make more intense interactions.

Children thus display unexpected abilities even in the very early stages of infancy. Sometimes this is elicited subconsciously, as soon as parents create the necessary preconditions and supplement the child's behavioural capabilities. So, while carrying your baby, particularly sitting on your hip, he also has the opportunity to independently turn towards the source of the environmental stimuli that meets his momentary needs and accomplishments, even when he cannot yet stabilise his head. By clinging to your body and gently lifting and turning his head he can independently make eye contact with you or direct his interest to the environment around him. If tired, he can turn his head on his own initiative away to your body. This is an unexpected achievement and signifies an independent choice to move away from anything that is too much. Not without good reason does Jean Liedloff describe being carried as an experience for the infant 'which prepares him for further development in the direction of self-responsibility'.[74] And don't forget: as mentioned before, carried babies can stabilise their head earlier due to the training effect (see page 71).

When a baby is carried he is involved in all events, but he is by no means the focus of them. He also takes part in the activities from the same viewing height as the adults and experiences other people who are not just 'standing over him'. He gets to know the interaction partners from an equal perspective, 'at eye level'. To feel the familiar caregiver in close proximity means that he can explore the environment from a tangible, secure base. Two components are always inherent in the new and unknown: it is interesting and requires exploration, but it can also be unpredictable and dangerous and must be considered with caution. In a settled atmosphere new things lose their uncertain or even threatening components and stimulate exploratory behaviour. Over the next few years too, this is overwhelmingly dependent on the current familiar reference person. An extra glance at the mother's face to seek assurance, when her features signal the 'safety' of the situation, encourages the curious explorer and gives the infant guidance in a situation he has not previously been able to assess. A sceptical reaction from the caregiver causes fear in the child

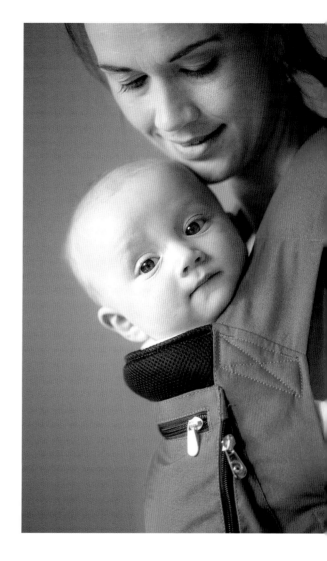

– and an anxious, more suspicious facial expression from the parent has a more lasting effect than the expression of joy.[75] **To be closely wrapped against the body of a familiar caregiver is the best starting position for approaching strange people or new objects – although this is 'just' a good precondition and not a guarantee that the child will respond positively to** **the unfamiliar stimulus.** When visiting the grandparents for the first time, mum and dad can beam at grandfather, but their offspring may still start to cry on seeing the beard or the bushy eyebrows – even though it may later become one of his greatest pleasures to pull granddad's beard. As an inexperienced little boy, he must first get used to a lot of things.

An upright body position encourages the attentiveness of a newborn, who then, if held correctly and securely, can show unexpected patterns of physical activity, even at this early stage. When being carried he can independently address the environmental stimuli that correspond to his momentary needs, or turn away from them if it is too much.

Closeness and distance – the development of independence

Parental sensitivity is closely related to many positive behavioural aspects of infants. In the classic investigations of attachment behaviour, six- to nine-month-old babies with more sensitive mothers cried less and were less likely to react in a fretful, aggressive or anxious way later. They trusted the mother's availability and willingness to help. **They looked for closeness when distressed but released themselves when they were comforted.** Overall they showed an equal balance between independent play and joy on having contact with their mother.[76] I do not want to discriminate against fathers in any way, but these classic studies were primarily carried out with mothers, they are usually the principal attachment figures. A child will build his own relationship with his father and can readily have a secure relationship with him, even if the child has an insecure relationship with the mother.

Even though the arguments in favour of the parent–child relationship usually focus on the development of the child, we should remind ourselves that as parents we also get something out of the emotional connection between us and the child. We gain more than just a more content and settled baby. Our initial readiness to respond and

cooperate is 'rewarded' even after the end of the first year of life as the toddler is more responsive to instructions, commands and prohibitions and is more likely to observe them.[77] The wording used above 'They looked for closeness when distressed but released themselves when they were comforted.' shows an equal balance between independent play and joy on having contact, and suggests that **children who are sure of the protection of their**

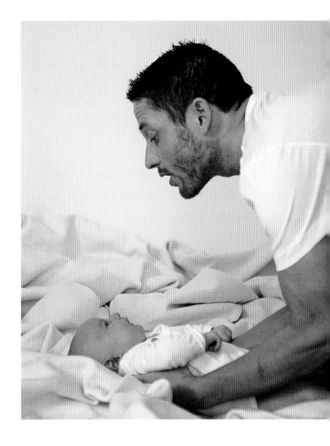

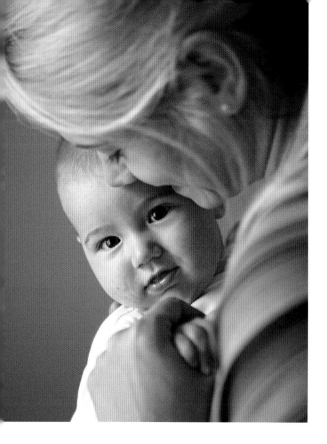

pendently for longer periods of time. The fears that babies who enjoy close physical contact in their first months of life through being carried will not be ready to give up this closeness at the appropriate time and will become too clingy are unfounded. The idea contradicts the results of the attachment research. The behaviour of the baby is not dependent on whether or not he is carried; it is the quality of the attachment he has with his parent that matters most.[79] As the research conducted by Anisfeld proved, carried children more often develop a secure attachment, since the intensive closeness created by carrying enables the parents to better respond to their baby.

Observations of different societies also back this up. In cultures such as the !Kung bush people of the South African steppe, for example, there is very close contact between the parents and the child during babyhood. However, in contrast, after babyhood, the !Kung children distance themselves further from their mothers than children of the same age in the UK. The initial constant closeness in no way results in the feared dependence of the children on the mother.[80] The American doctor and anthropologist, Melvin J. Konner,[81] concludes that because babies initially have such frequent physical contact, they find it easy to remove themselves from their mothers, to explore the environment independently and seek

parents and consider them to be the safety net in all stressful situations develop greater independence and are more confident. After all, from this firm foundation, a child can take a few risks. The child is more likely to venture out and display exploratory behaviour, rather than fearful reticence, if he feels secure.[78] Securely attached children are more socially competent and respond to other people appropriately for their age; they are less irritable and, even at a young age, demonstrate that they can play inde-

out others to interact with. Of course, other factors in addition to carrying and physical contact are bound to play a part. In these cultures, set against the protective parental back-ground, children have positive experiences with more than one or two familiar adults, as well as other, older children, even during infancy. In addition, they are constantly integrated in mixed-age groups of children from a young age.[82] Physical closeness and carrying in traditional cultures are indications of a fundamentally different approach to childcare. It remains to be seen to what extent this can be carried over into our culture. However, the trend in many Western societies of bringing up children for early independence – so that they fall asleep alone, play alone, lie alone in the rocker, occupy themselves independently so that family life isn't too interrupted, in other words, 'not spoiling them' – actually leads to the opposite of what the parents are trying so hard to achieve. Thus the educational goal of 'early autonomy' often leads to 'early insecurity'.[83]

A secure attachment to their parents allows children to explore their environment in a competent manner from an early age. Being confident of their relationship with their parents means that they can give up the closeness to their mother and father independently and expand their range of behaviour. By the end of their first year of age, closely attached children are more likely to react to and follow instructions from their parents. Parents thus also benefit from their early emotional input.

Babywearing in special situations

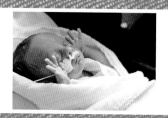

Premature babies – a break from the incubator

Physical contact and closeness are important for a baby and promote development. If this applies to children who experience normal development, how much more significant is this aspect for very small babies who haven't had a normal start in life? Observations of premature babies have already been mentioned in various chapters, particularly with regard to intensive skin stimulation and perception of movement (see, for example, page 62), which also resulted in babies being able to leave hospital earlier. Hammocks or gently moving waterbeds encourage more regular breathing, optimum cardiac activity and also improve muscle tone. Enhanced stomach and intestinal function was also observed as part of a highly complex range of benefits.[84] Premature babies who also received additional 'touch stimulation'

perceived their environment in a more intensive way, oriented and controlled themselves and their feelings better, settled quicker, were less irritable and cried less, having an improved ability to self-regulate. Follow-up investigations at home confirmed that their overall development was more satisfactory. Physical problems occurred less often than is normal for premature babies. It was also significant that these infants were better accepted by their parents than children who didn't benefit from these massage sessions.[85]

Luckily, the understanding that the best 'therapy' for prematurity is intensive physical contact between the parents and the baby is now widespread. With the kangaroo method, premature babies are laid directly in skin-to-skin contact on the chest of the parent as often as possible – as soon as their condition allows it – and a blanket is put over them. In this way babies are kept warm and safe. The method originated out of necessity. Due to a lack of incubators in a clinic in Bogota, Columbia, the body heat of the mother was used to stabilise the temperature of babies born too early. The mortality rate of children cared for in this way was significantly lower than that of the babies remaining in the incubators, even though some had been born extremely early. Even if this success must be taken into account against the background of bad conditions in an overcrowded, poorly equipped hospital that cannot be compared to general standards in European clinics, the results were nevertheless ground breaking.[86] Subsequent research showed in ever more detail how important this form of physical closeness is for the overall development of a premature baby, even for those with the very low body weight of just over 700 grams (1lb 8oz), born just after the 25th week of pregnancy.[87] **The 'kangaroo care method' moved the small world of the premature baby closer to his original environment in the uterus, which bears no comparison with the isolated existence in an incubator.**

If babies are able to enjoy the benefits of the kangaroo method, these tiny, delicate infants can stabilise themselves more quickly without the use of an incubator, and they are kept warm thanks to the body temperature of the adult. They soon establish a regular heartbeat and breathing frequency that are within the optimum range. Their sleep is deeper, and when awake, they are more frequently in a peaceful alert state. Their weight gain is also greater. As a result, they are able to leave the incubator earlier and thus ultimately be discharged from the clinic earlier than babies who have not been carried on the mother's chest.[88] Kangaroo care is important for both the parents and their tiny babies. As well as making physical contact through the closeness of carrying, the parents can also make gentle emotional contact with their babies. It is striking that mothers and fathers also often subsequently unconsciously adopt the typical stroking pattern that is generally characteristic of initial contact directly after birth. Just a little instruction and encouragement

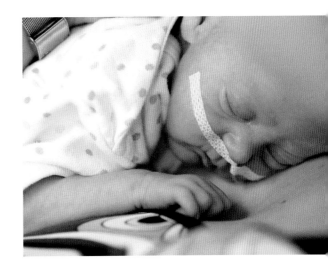

during the first physical contact is sometimes enough for the parents to feel confident in handling such a delicate being. **The more frequently they feel their child directly, the more familiarity they gain and the more they can develop an emotional relationship.**[89] This is an important remark. With premature births there is always a great risk that parents will have difficulty developing this emotional relationship with a baby who doesn't look as they 'expected'. On the one hand the period immediately after the birth follows a

routine, and, due to the physiological instability of the premature baby, there is no opportunity to create physical and emotional closeness. On the other hand parents also have to overcome the problem of the premature birth and also miss out on the usual circumstances of birth with all its ups and downs. Parents are often unable to handle their delicate and fragile-looking baby normally for weeks on end.[90] And even when they can finally take their baby in their arms, their actions are inhibited and they hardly dare to stroke him. Due to the long separation caused by the initial hospital stay, they find it hard to form an emotional relationship. Worries about the child's physical development in the long-term take centre stage. As a result of all these difficult circumstances, premature babies are comparatively often the victims of child abuse, due to a lack of emotional closeness. In contrast to this are the fascinating scenes observed when even extremely premature babies are nestled against the chest of their mother or father, escaping from the incubator for a short time and making contact with their parents, and vice versa.

Premature babies who experience skin-to-skin contact using the kangaroo method develop better overall and can usually be discharged from hospital earlier. Physical contact and perception of movement do more than just calm – they also have a positive effect on breathing, cardiac activity and the child's muscle tone.

Special needs children – not an easy start to life

It is not only premature babies who have trouble getting love and affection from their parents. Children who are disabled in any way have a different starting point in comparison with normally developed children and thus have special requirements. They experience a lack of support at another level (due to the difficulties in winning parental affection), which has an additional negative effect on their development. Their 'strengths' are now linked to the area of emotions and are thus unavailable for overcoming their special problem areas. To put it another way: **if disabled children are also supported in the areas outside of their problem area, their additional strengths are released, and they are probably more likely to master their disability.** Like other children, disabled children generally benefit from being carried as this satisfies their basic need for closeness and physical contact and they also receive additional motor support due to the stimulation of different senses with the associated parts of the brain.

However, with some disabilities, the problem initially lies with the parents, who have great difficulties when the child does not match the image they had of him during pregnancy. Premature babies or

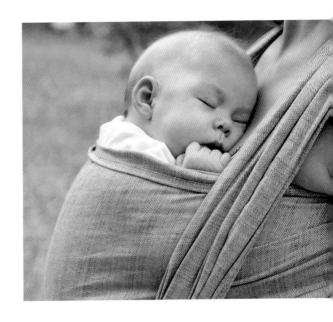

very delicate newborns lack the familiar 'baby fat' which is so appealing to us and which is only formed – if at all – during the final weeks before birth. The familiar baby face, which has such a wonderful effect on the 'childcare start button', is not there. Even this deviation from the required image sometimes causes parents to have difficulties addressing their little one emotionally. The same applies even more so for children who present with mal-formations at birth. In particular, if these affect the neck, head or facial area, they can have serious repercussions. For example, a cleft lip and jaw often present a major emotional obstacle for parents and here physical closeness is even more important as it can be the precursor for the development of the emotional parental bond. And don't forget: carrying in a sling, wrap or carrier also offers 'protection from the outside world' for fathers and mothers. For unsure, highly sensitive parents, the bemused looks of passers-by – after the initial curious look into the pushchair – are almost unbearable. Carrying their baby all snuggled up in a wrap protects them from inquisitive looks, simplifies the normal everyday life of the parents and makes the regular stroll more bearable, so they don't have to run the gauntlet of explanations or sympathetic looks.[91]

Parents of children with Down's Syndrome often need this protection at first until they have recovered their emotional stability and have developed inner protection against significant looks from the outside world. However, the diminished muscle tone of children disabled in this way often puts parents off carrying the child at first. **Children with developmental problems, however, profit particularly well from the varied stimuli offered by being carried.** All senses are stimulated, and by being securely and tightly fastened, the baby is freed from the task of stabilising his body and can address other external stimuli.

When carrying a baby with diminished muscle tone, particular attention must be paid to a good tying technique.

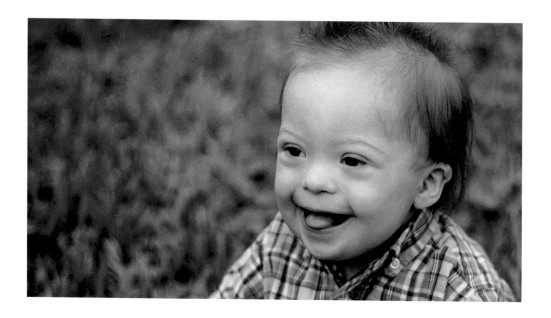

The body of a baby with Down's Syndrome needs intensive support for much longer than is otherwise required. On the other hand, the constant small physical balancing movements in the sling or wrap caused by the movement of the parent create a training effect that a baby in a pushchair would miss out on. Of course, in the case of a Down's Syndrome baby there are no general recommendations on how a child should best be tied in the wrap.[92] The factors that must be taken into account are too varied. Cooperation with the appropriate trained therapists, babywearing educators and doctors is essential.

Disabled children, and their parents, benefit from babywearing. On the one hand, it is one of the best chances to create an emotional relationship through closeness, and on the other parents need this emotional protection until they have found their inner stability.

When something goes wrong – babies with asymmetries

If a baby has to 'fight' against a lateral curve in the spine – scoliosis – this can be due to several factors. In most cases, asymmetries of the spine in babies are caused by an intrauterine predicament. During the first year of life, they generally re-form spontaneously and completely.[93] Sometimes babies' spines realign as soon as they are carried upright. **The choice of carrying position, for example, favouring one side or the other, can consciously work against asymmetries in a targeted way.**

In the case of asymmetric posture or a tendency to a flattened head, upright carrying has also proved to be an option for moving babies from their preferred sleep position and counteracting the condition.

There is another way in which babywearing can, at least partially, have a positive effect on the baby's body. Positional plagiocephaly (flattening of the head) has become more frequent in recent years as babies are primarily laid down on their backs to sleep to prevent sudden infant death syndrome (SIDS). According to an overview study, around 22 per cent of newborns had this condition. Even though this flattening often disappears again during the first two years of life, in more severe cases it can cause further problems and pathological developments. So from a medical perspective it appears increasingly important to start countermeasures early.[94] One approach is to move the baby from the horizontal position whenever possible during daytime sleep. Unsurprisingly, parents can do this most easily and in the most satisfactory way for both parties by carrying their baby upright in a wrap.

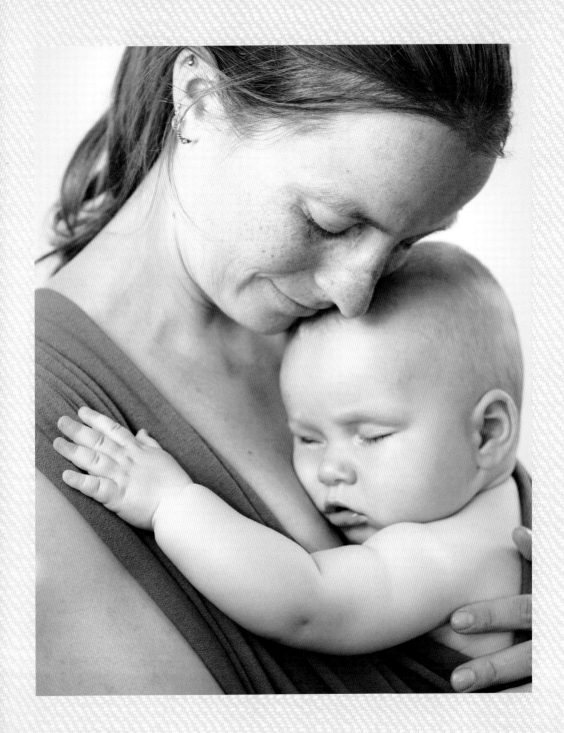

Please, no stereotypes!

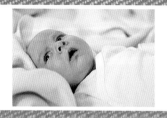

Perhaps this discussion of babywearing has confirmed your initial ideas and you just need one last confirmation. Or maybe you need more black and white arguments to use against the ever more frequent warning voices from all around you. Perhaps you were unsure, had some doubts and needed information to be able to finally decide whether and how you should carry your baby. Now, convinced, you have bought a suitable soft carrier – and have packed your baby in to it. You might have been fortunate to have a passionate sling or wrap user or babywearing educator to introduce you to the correct tying techniques. Or your midwife might have shown you all the little tricks, and **you are fine with this straight away:** *Exhilarated, you set off, your baby enjoys the physical closeness, as do you – and you also enjoy your new freedom.*

No more switching between everyday tasks and the fussy baby with his justified claims for closeness. Now the sweet little bundle of joy sits in the wrap, sometimes he falls asleep straight away or else he watches your activities with interest; sometimes he also gets involved. Many parents have since learned the extent to which their readiness to carry their baby can facilitate everyday life and they have described it on the internet. The needs of an infant turn your daily schedule upside down, planning is an unachievable illusion, and it's all about successful coordination and sometimes even disaster management. By having the baby in the wrap it is a lot easier to accommodate his sudden needs for contact. Not everything can or should revolve around the baby – you also have justified requirements during the daily routine, along with the rest of the family. This means that reasonable compromises have to be found for all participants. Although we always talk about the wonderful interaction between parent and baby while carrying, you must still do the dishes, peel the potatoes and cook the dinner. And at this point, the baby starts to squawk piteously. Placing him quickly on your back in a wrap is always better than listening to his complaints from the crib or the pushchair, or trying to wash the plates, pots and knives in a rush, or even delaying the mountain of tasks until the dear little one has a rare nap – just about holding onto the limit of what is bearable. Take a moment to think which means of carrying him would be best for all concerned, not just for your baby. You don't love him any less when you also think about yourself. Even if all this fuss is not ideal, you are still giving him something important: your closeness.

Maybe your experience of carrying is rather different. *Exhilarated, you set off, your baby is enjoying the physical closeness and so are you – for a while.* After fifteen minutes, your back begins to ache. You check the position of the wrap or the soft carrier, which all of a sudden is not quite so comfortable and simply hurts and causes muscle tension. You ask your friend – an enthusiastic babywearer – for advice and you also ask your midwife. Nothing helps. After carrying for a maximum of thirty minutes, you regularly have to give

up, exhausted and somewhat confused. You can feel the pain in your back for a long time afterwards and your shoulders are tense. You just wanted to give your baby as much physical closeness as possible. Your guilty conscience grows because, after all, you are depriving your child of varied experiences. Don't worry about either – you don't need to carry the baby for hours at a time, nor do you need a guilty conscience! Your baby is hardly likely to cuddle up and enjoy the closeness when your muscles are tense and hard. The only thing to consider in such a situation is whether there might be a

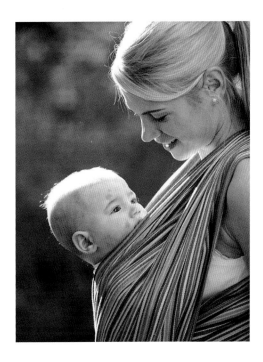

different way of carrying your baby that is more suited to your body. Maybe it would be better to carry him on your back, or perhaps you should switch to an ergonomically balanced, comfortable, soft-structured carrier, to a Mei Tai or, more likely the reverse, from one of these to a more basic sling or woven wrap. If this doesn't help either and you can only manage to carry your baby for ten or twenty minutes without discomfort, then stop at ten or twenty minutes. You can still give your baby important experiences in this short time. Every minute counts, even if the pushchair takes over for extended walks. Look at it like this: Daddy

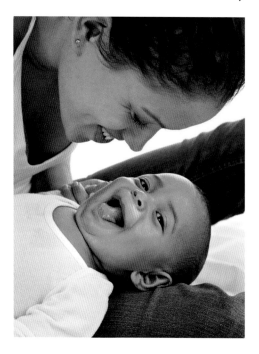

can finally do something that you can't, and both of you will enjoy the long walks just as much. To give some comfort, in the scientific research that showed that carried babies are more often securely attached, the parents carried their children for an average of just thirty minutes per day, and sometimes not on every day (see page 80).

Some mothers who experienced pain when carrying their babies were found to have spinal damage or other posturural complaints. If this applies to you, it may be worth visiting your doctor. Another factor to consider is whether or not you started to carry at too late a stage. If your child was already a little older (and hence heavier) when you began, you will have missed out on the automatic training effect that occurs if you carry your baby from the start.

There is another possible situation. *Exhilarated, you set off. Your baby enjoys the physical closeness, as do you. You don't want to deprive your friend and her child of this experience.* She had a difficult birth with a Caesarean section and the little one had to stay in hospital for a while. Intense physical contact can only be a good thing! In spite of all your efforts, your friend is not particularly keen on babywearing. You offer her a wrap – but she doesn't get on with it. You buy her a good carrier –

but after a while you find out that it remains unused in the cupboard. You have made so much effort to convince your friend how important carrying is for the parent–child relationship, all to no avail. You press the point and finally your friend replies that she finds it unbearably constricting. She doesn't find the closeness to her child enriching and sees it as rather unpleasant and tiring. Just leave it at that. Your friend has not found babywearing and the associated close physical contact with her child as wonderful as you, in fact she sees it as a negative thing. In the long term, it is not particularly good for the mother–child relationship if babywearing becomes forced, whether due to the persuasiveness of a good friend or the mother's own rational considerations after reading about the positive effects and thus feeling obliged to carry her baby.

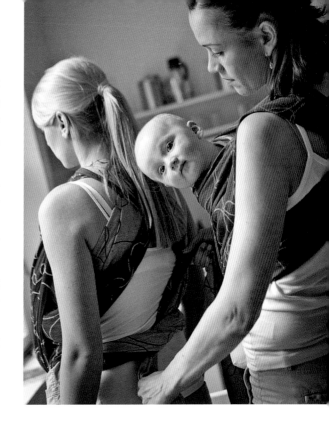

Obligatory carrying will tend to harm the development of the emotional relationship between the mother and child more than support it, if internal rejection remains after the initial attempts. This defeats the object. Physical contact and closeness should be seen as positive for all parties concerned; only then can all the points described over the last pages develop. The experiences of an infant being carried are unique in terms of the combination of sensory stimulation. If they are carried in arms without assistance, carrying times are mostly very restricted. The issue then becomes one of offering the baby sensory stimulation in other ways wherever possible. Although this requires significantly greater effort on the parent's side, it is possible.

Varied, fun, movement games are necessary to give experience of movement. Physical contact can be provided by intensive periods of interaction, regular baby massages, extended cuddle time and small stroking actions. This might be of no great consequence if your baby needs comparatively little physical closeness for his satisfaction. Every child is different, but each needs some degree of closeness. And if you cannot provide the carrying option yourself, maybe another family member could do so – cede some ground to the enthusiastic daddy for once. A mother doesn't have to be able to do everything. Ideology is out of place here.

Another possible scenario. *You have bought a wonderful wrap and taken a course on how to use it correctly – but your baby doesn't want to be carried.* The few cases I know of directly are probably due to the fact the children were almost six months old when the mothers first attempted to

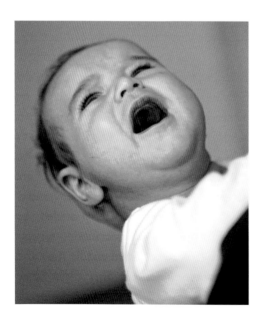

carry them. It cannot be completely ruled out that, when carrying is commenced later, the unease of the parent also plays a role that is reflected in refusal by the children. There are so many examples from other areas in which the unease of the parents is transferred to their children. However, the close constriction can irritate a baby who is unused to this and he could find it unpleasant and fight against it. By contrast, a newborn will see the confinement of the wrap as something familiar from his time in the uterus. Being wrapped up returns him to the security of this period. Babies obviously notice the insecurity and awkwardness of their parents during initial attempts at carrying, but it does not seem to harm them in any way in the long term. When parents choose to carry, many of them carry their babies during the first weeks of life and – according to one long-term study – more than half of the babies had their 'introduction to carrying' within the first three weeks of life.[95] Only a few parents reported that their babies regularly protested against being packed into a sling, wrap or other carrier at the beginning, even though all that was usually needed was a few knee bends and steps to swing the baby's mood from displeasure to visible ease. However, if your child should continue to reject the carrier, there are still the above options for providing physical closeness and experience of movement – without a guilty conscience on your part!

Being carried is neither an essential precondition nor a guarantee for the successful development of a baby or a positive parent–child relationship – but it is a good foundation for it. You should not force yourself to carry your child for hours each day if you do not feel comfortable doing it, nor ignore the needs of your baby for independent activities in the belief that carrying is, in principle, good for your child. He needs regular physical contact with you but also sufficient opportunity for independent experiences. Times in which he can explore his own body, practice his skills and investigate different objects are just as important for his development as closeness to you. When, how long, and how often is dependent on the child's age as well as the individual characteristics of your baby. Anyone who thinks that they can give firm guidelines on this is exceeding their competence – and underestimating that of the parents and their children who, if they are in tune with each other and responsive, can perceive and signal which activities are required. This calls for sensitivity on the part of the parents.

Good parents, bad parents, good childhood, bad childhood: this doesn't necessarily have anything to do with whether or not parents carry their babies – even though, at first glance, this sentence appears to question everything that has been described in this book. Those who prefer pushchairs and those who prefer babywearing all want to be good parents and give their baby the best start in life – those who carry their baby are convinced that they are doing the right thing and so are those who use pushchairs. So sometimes, using a sling or wrap also seems to demonstrate a particular philosophy of life. This may be true for some parents as they want to adjust their life to the needs of the child – there is no problem with this. With others, it is only due to reasons of practicality and well-being. This is also OK and significantly facilitates family life. However, sometimes there is more behind the wrap. It seems that parental love is 'leased' with the wrap, and of course this isn't the case. Others suspect that behind the 'piece of material', as the ethnologist Timo Heimerdinger so strikingly describes it, the woman as a mother is now tied to the baby with the wrap instead of being tied to the oven. They believe that through her love for the child she is seduced into self-abandonment as in earlier times – and they consider the achievements of the women's movement to be at risk.[96] Given this assumption, fathers who carry their offspring in a wrap or other carrier emerge as a glimmer of light on the horizon. However you see this discussion, it becomes critical when a judgement is made based on the act of carrying, the type of carrying and even the tying method. **Information is good, but judgements have no place here, except in situations in which the quality or design of the sling or carrier may endanger the child's health.** It would be good if the discussion of babywearing was only confined to what best suits parents and their child as a two- or three-person team. It would also be nice if carrying were to become a generally accepted care technique, just like using a pushchair. If both could stand on an equal footing – something that some parents have been putting into practice in their everyday life for a long time – without displaying any ideological characteristics to the world, this would mean that parents could simply make a choice based on what is right and important to them. It would carry the same weight as the fact that you might

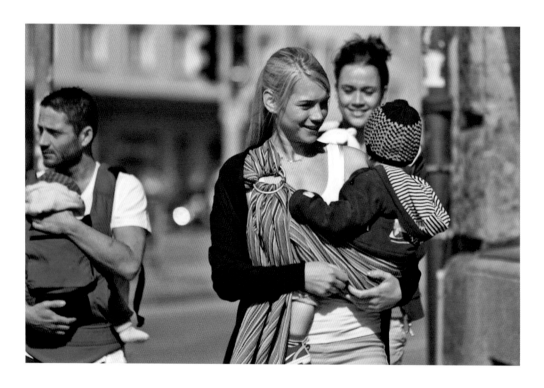

decide to take part in a baby swimming or baby massage course, to purchase this or the other child seat, or decide on a blue or green romper suit – or not.

Being carried is not a requirement or a guarantee for a successful parent–child relationship, even though it is a good foundation for it.

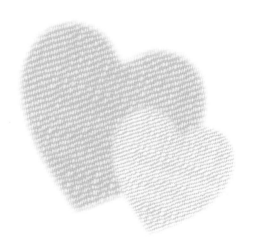

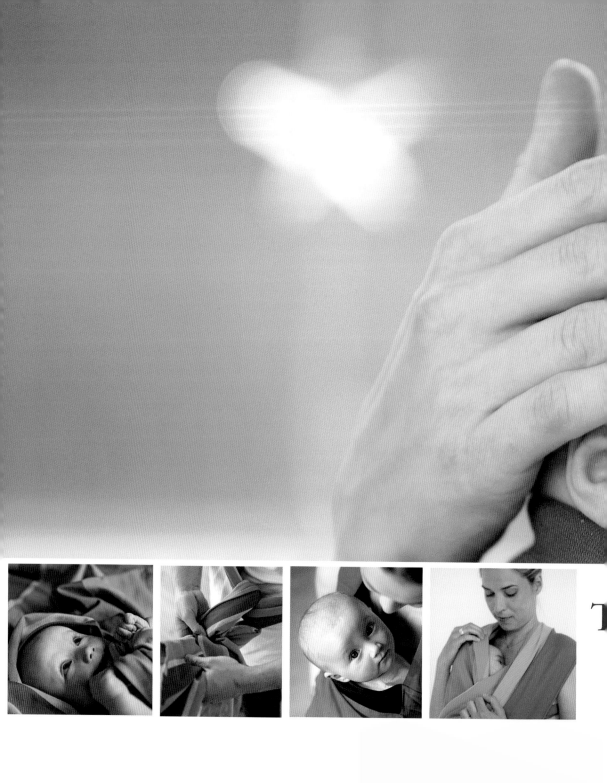

T

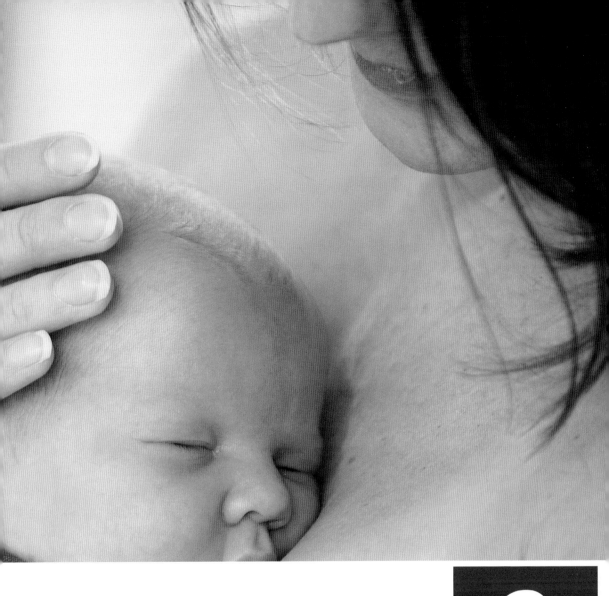

practicalities of babywearing:
how to carry your child

2

The big question: which carrier and which way of carrying?

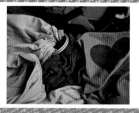

Babywearing isn't just carrying

In the first part of the book we saw that:

- carrying encourages the motor, sensory and cognitive development of your baby
- it helps to develop a child's self-confidence and his social and other skills
- it supports a good parent–child relationship
- you also benefit from the carrying experience
- it does not cause postural damage to your child.

Now we finally get to the point: what is the best way to carry your baby? In a wrap or a sling, in a pouch or a ring sling, in a kangaroo carrier, a soft structured carrier or in something else?

Whatever you choose, the basic requirements remain the same. The first requirement is the same for all options: it must be suitable for the anatomical and physiological characteristics of a baby at *any* age, *any* size and *any* weight.

The earlier common reservations against carrying a baby in an upright position were not completely without justification given the carriers available at this time. **There were – and are – carrying methods and carriers on the market that are unsuitable or which do not meet the requirements that should be placed upon them.** Specifically this means that they do not adequately support a baby in the spinal area and/or do not guarantee an optimum leg position. Most children can certainly cope with a less than optimum position, and in the course of their development ultimately compensate for anything lacking – at least if the circumstances do not differ too greatly from the requirements and the individual characteristics of the child. But why should you be satisfied with a less-than-perfect solution when there are better options available? Demand the highest standards – they are justified and you are justified in demanding them. After all, you are the responsible parent or carer.

By clarifying whether or not you want to use a wrap, another wrap-like variant or a different type of baby carrier, you are already on the right track. This leads us to the next point: which wrap and tying method, or which sling or carrier to choose from all those found on the market? Not every tying technique is suitable for every age, and the structure of the fabric of some wraps makes tying unnecessarily difficult. Not every available carrier is equally suitable or fit for purpose. The range of wraps and other carriers on the market is confusing for newcomers. And you can't always rely on advice from baby equipment retailers. Here, it is often the design and brand name rather than the quality that determines which product is sold and recommended. And, in addition, more and more carriers are available on the internet. Enthusiastic comments from users are also immediately available. International products – many from the USA – are easy to obtain, but, they must be considered with a particularly critical eye as the manufacturers frequently focus on different criteria than in regions that can boast a longer 'modern' tradition of babywearing (such as in some European countries). The whole topic is complex. If you choose an unsuitable carrier, you are not doing yourself or your baby any favours. If your rock-hard muscles are screaming after a short time carrying, you will not be able to summon up any enthusiasm for carrying your baby or be able to enjoy his closeness. If you feel that your child is sliding out of the wrap, sling or carrier, or if he is not sitting in a stable position, your purchase will soon lead a forgotten existence in a corner. It isn't easy, but you should do a lot of research, just as you do before you purchase a child car seat.

Nowadays you can access up-to-date consumer tests in magazines and also find information on the internet. It goes without saying that hazardous materials must not be used in any areas a child may come into

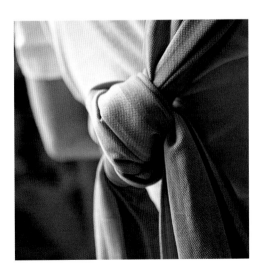

direct skin contact with – especially with their face and mouth. Everyone must judge for themselves how important it is to ensure that there is no bleach in the brand labels or traces of unwanted materials in inaccessible areas or threads. However, looking at the tests, you should pay attention to the individual assessment criteria and not just look at the final assessment. For example, the less-than-perfect body position of your baby is a far more important criterion than unhelpful instructions. They could be found on the internet or somewhere else.

If you prefer a more hands-on approach, there are many sling libraries which allow you to try baby carriers before you buy. Search the internet for one local to you.

How long and from when?

Babywearing should not be a chore or based on the number of hours to be completed per day. It is a question of the age and the individual peculiarities of the mother and child. Some babies are more in need of love and require more physical proximity. A baby may also want to be carried more today and less tomorrow. If something unusual happens or if an unsettling burst of development takes place, the baby might constantly need your closeness one day. The next day he may be more settled and prefer to be alone or play on his own and have his own physical experiences. Trust your feeling of what he prefers. When the baby starts to toddle, carrying is reduced almost automatically as the floor is now the adventure playground on which he can move about under his own steam.

If you are wondering when to start carrying, there is only one recommendation: when you and your baby feel comfortable and when you have found a carrying method you feel confident with. You can carry your baby in an upright position from the start. The earlier you start to carry, the earlier you and your baby can enjoy and use the advantages of intensive closeness, but you must both feel really comfortable.

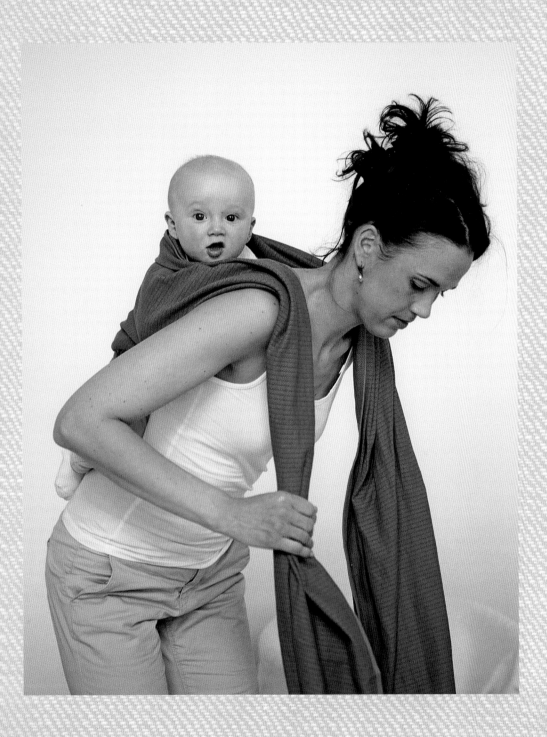

The essentials for carrying your baby upright: the correct position

Initially I would like to summarise the points that are necessary for a good position in a sling, a wrap or another carrier when you are carrying your baby in an upright position, regardless of whether on the front, the hip or the back. **The following basic points should help you decide whether you have tied your baby correctly in a wrap or whether the carrier you want to use is even suitable.** Although the following guidelines refer to soft carriers and not explicitly to wraps – this would only lead to complicated explanations – a child should be tied into a wrap in the same way as the instructions given here for other carriers.

- **The child's leg position** The legs should be tucked up at least to a right angle, ideally up to 100 or 110° – a squat position is particularly important for newborns and during the first three to four months. The carrier should be set up so that it secures the tucked leg position (see the chapter on hip dysplasia and carrying from page 42). This is only the case when the base of the carrier located under the bottom of the baby and between the thighs is wide enough to reach from the hollow of the knee to the other (see Fig.

10, page 119). The stretching of the legs can also be prevented in another way – with an overbag. The instructions always state that the hollows of the knees should be higher than the nappy and this also applies for the different types of carriers. The carriers that are 'baggy' in the nappy area best meet this requirement. After all, your baby tends to sit in a thick nappy. To ensure that his bottom is then lower than the backs of the knees, there must be enough room for the nappy and the baby's bottom, otherwise his legs may not be tucked up enough.

At this point it becomes clear that carrying a baby facing outward so that he isn't looking at you cannot in any way support the correct leg position. Even though some manufacturers of carriers advertise this position, it is not a suitable position for the baby. More on this subject can be found on page 170.

- **Adequate support for the child's back** When a baby cannot sit upright independently, it is particularly important that the back part of the carrier tightly encloses the child and supports him in such a way that he is upright and not tilted to the side in the carrier or slumped over. This usually implies that the baby is closely snuggled into the mother. But even when a child can sit safely by him-self, he should not collapse when asleep, so even when he's older he still needs the support and stability of the body of the person carrying him.

- **Head support.** The rear part of the carrying aid should, if possible, extend above the baby's head and also offer lateral support so that the head does not roll around without control. This is particularly important in the first weeks of life as a baby does not yet have sufficient control of his head. But even later, the support is still needed during sleep.

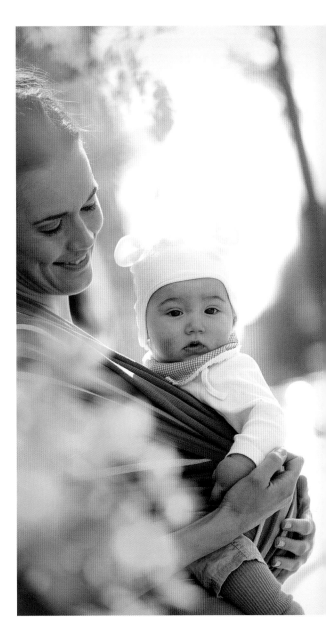

To help you decide

You should always check these three points, with any type of carrier or method of tying a wrap. If you want to purchase a carrier, don't forget that your baby will grow quickly. It should be possible to adjust the carrier to his physical circumstances throughout the whole period in which you want to carry your baby, so make sure he has enough room to grow or you will soon have to buy a new one. Some manufacturers even offer newborn inserts for their products to extend the suitability of the carrier to the very small. The outcome of this may be suitable for anatomical requirements, but convenience often leaves much to be desired and/or it is difficult to use. Or it doesn't fit during an 'in-between period'. You don't face this problem if you choose a wrap. A wrap can 'grow' constantly and the tying methods can vary according to age, although initially you must decide on the length of the material, so you should already have a rough idea of which wrap and tying method you plan to use. The location on the body is most variable with a wrap, though some carriers allow different locations too. And for you as the babywearer, the strain placed by the weight of your baby is minimised when he is snuggled closely into your body – a plus point for a wrap or a carrier such as a ring sling. On the other hand, today there are ergonomic carriers that transfer the weight of the child partly to the hip area of the person carrying and thus relieve the back and shoulder area. For anyone whose back is a problem area, a carrier of this type may be better – particularly given the increasing weight of your bouncing baby.

Ultimately, the proof of the pudding is in the eating. One type of carrier may be perfect for your friend and her baby, but it may not suit your anatomy or the proportions of your little one. Midwives, parenting centres, babywearing educators and others sometimes have a good selection of different carriers for you to try on or borrow. Babywearing meetings, slingmeets or classes will offer you the best chance to try out a range of wraps, carriers and slings and to learn about them. Some manufacturers, businesses and online retailers also approach their customers and provide products to try out or take them back if they don't suit.

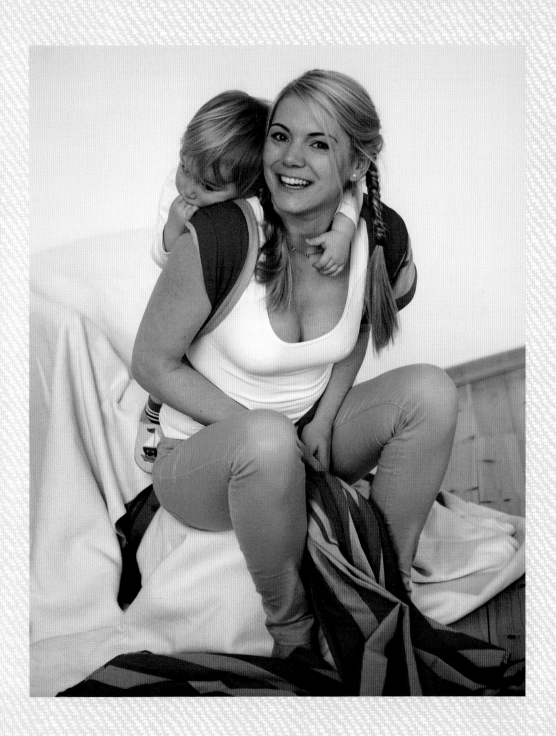

Soft structured carriers

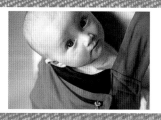

Special features
- Easy to use.
- A good soft structured carrier takes into account the anatomy of the child.
- Some carriers transfer part of the baby's weight via a waist band to the hip of the person carrying and thus relieve the back and shoulder areas.

Points to consider
- Some carriers are not recommended due to their design.
- The most frequent problem is that the perfect tuck position is not achieved. Only a few carriers allow the legs to bend at more than 90° and often the legs are even hanging down.
- Support in the back area is often not sufficient.

With most designs, the children are carried in front of the chest, in the face-to-face position. Sometimes a 'rucksack carrying method' is possible, but the right hip position is rarely feasible. The greater the number of carrying options, the more complicated it becomes to achieve success.

Even novices can usually get on with most carriers immediately and this is an advantage. However, the carrier available in stores must – as mentioned above – be carefully examined, as a lot of them do not take the child's anatomy into account at all. Some manufacturers try to encourage carrying facing outward and these should be avoided. More on page 170.

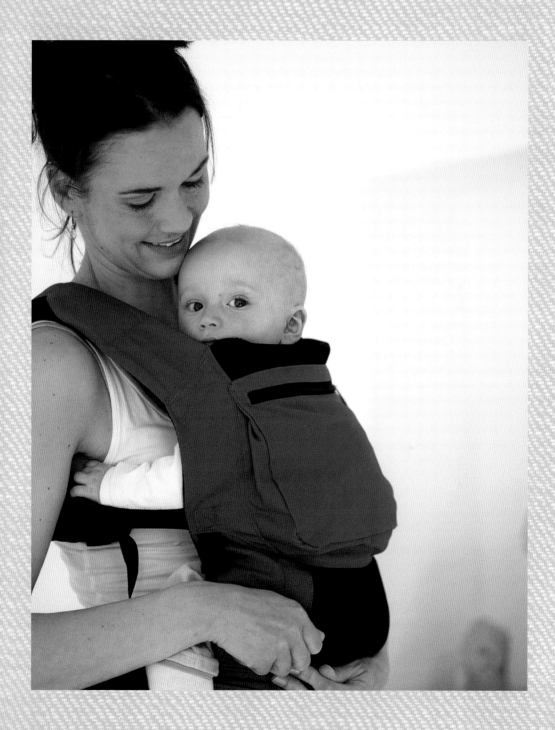

What should parents look for when buying a carrier?

The first thing you should look at is the leg position your child would assume in the carrier and you will then be able to rule out several of the carriers as unsuitable. You can also look at the product images from the manufacturer on the internet. **If the base part between the legs is too narrow and does not reach from the hollow of one knee to that of the other when the legs are** *tucked***, the legs will hang down more or less extended in the hip joints.** The same applies for a base part made of soft material that can be easily squashed. And the little rascals will certainly do this when they become more agile.

The recommendation to research the suitability of different carriers is important, but you may not find examples of all types of carrier. Only a selection are tested, although the most common products are often included. Sometimes a test isn't even necessary as it is sufficient to look at the advertising images to see the construction of the carrier. It is striking that some models unintentionally grip the backs of the baby's knees to force the tucked position. The manufacturer's web pages should give you at least some information about the suitability of their products.

Of course, it's always best to try out the carrier with your baby. You can't always find what you want among your circle of friends and advisors can't always help either. In this case, I believe that you should not be shy and should test the patience of retailers and sales people – after all, this concerns the health of your baby. And the efforts of some manufacturers or shops who offer, as previously mentioned, test products should be lauded. The internet can also help here.

Back to the list of deficiencies. **Sometimes the openings for the baby's legs are directed downwards.** In this case, a tucked thigh position is impossible and, with a face-to-face position, the infant's thighs are pushed into the body of the adult. Not only are the baby's legs hanging downwards due to not being in the squatting position, but the additional pressure on the thighs also increases the stretch in the hip joints, which actually encourages dysplasia instead of preventing or counteracting it.

It's hard to believe, but some designs are even worse and cause a more intense strain on the hip joints when the knees of the infant extend down to the thighs of the adult. This applies to carriers that cannot be adequately adjusted to the height of the parent, particularly to small, petite women, but sometimes the design itself is unsuitable even for people of average height. The baby simply hangs too low. The result is that with each step taken by the parent, the baby's knee is pushed back – from the perspective of the child. With each step the pressure on his thigh is increased. If this pressure and the stretch to the child's hip joints become too much, the baby can only get relief by changing the position of his pelvis. The pelvis is 'tipped down', which is automatically accompanied by a visible hollow back, an unnatural position for the spine in the first year of life. In this position, the shoulders and head of the baby fall backwards, a clear sign that the carrier is completely unsuitable.

Many carriers do not sufficiently support the baby's back. The pulling strength of the two straps that tighten the rear part of the carrier (Fig. 9, top right) are often the only support for the child's upper body. If there is also too much space between the person carrying and the baby, he can collapse completely unless the parents help and constantly support him with an arm.

A quick note on head supports. Some bend over backwards as soon as they are subject to gentle pressure. Others are placed too low or too far from the child from the outset to be a secure support for babies who cannot yet stabilise their head. They are often designed so that the head is not supported at the side and the baby can slump that way.

Some of the carriers even manage to

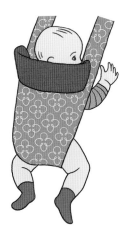

Fig. 9 Unsuitable: hanging legs. If the back can only remain steady through the pulling force of two straps, little babies quickly slump.

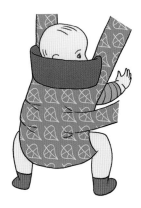

Fig. 10 Important: a wide and stable base. An additional stabilising method – for example a strap across the back – is important for tiny babies.

combine **all deficiencies.** I haven't mentioned the comfort of the carrier for the parent. Some carriers will be discarded on the first test – particularly when tried out with the child. Here the straps cannot be pulled tightly enough and there the buckle presses or something is cutting in. **The failings carry their own weight. You will soon notice them yourself.** As mentioned, the best thing is to borrow the baby carrier first and try it out with your baby.

Briefly: framed backpacks etc. are intended for older children who can already control their body and sit independently and safely for long periods. They are usually designed for children of nine months and older. Completely different assessment criteria apply to these carriers, which are not the focus of this discussion.

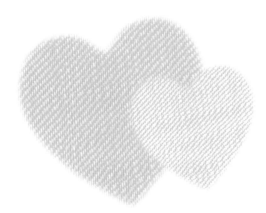

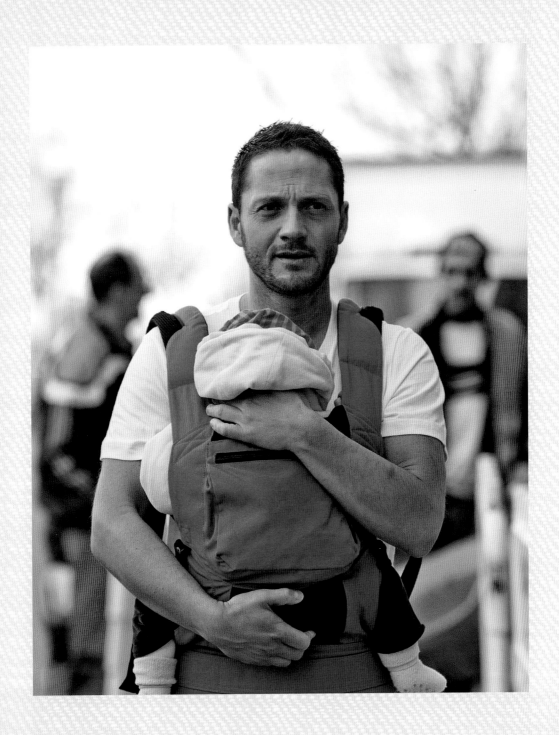

Using a woven wrap

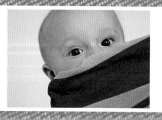

Special features

- Suitable for all ages; the wrap 'grows' with the child.
- Very versatile: to the front, on the back or on the hip, or even lying – all of these carrying positions are possible.
- As the baby is huddled closely to the person carrying him, the weight distribution is more favourable.

Points to consider

- Not everyone finds the tying techniques easy to learn.
- A certain degree of patience and practice is required so that the suitable tying techniques can be correctly executed.

Every beginning is hard

To ensure the correct leg position, to give the back the correct support, to support the head – and to do all this at the same time and also fight with the wrap, which is so incredibly long and voluminous, seems quite complicated. And when you first start learning to tie the wrap the baby seems tiny compared to the mountain of fabric and it is difficult to manoeuvre confidently. A basic introduction to the correct technique for tying the wrap would be very helpful for most parents – with the exception of a few gracious and talented self-teachers – so that carrying is not immediately discounted. Maybe you can learn the different tying techniques at an early stage and practise them by meeting with a babywearing educator or attending a babywearing class. This can make your life significantly easier. With a competent babywearing expert – nowadays there are even babywearing courses specifically for men – you can ask any questions that may be troubling you. You can learn which tying techniques are suitable for which age and why. You can also learn little tricks to help you get along with this piece of material, which can sometimes grow into a true monster.

Don't let your initial trials with the wrap degenerate into stress, either on your part or the baby's. A crying, stiff baby normally foils any attempt to use the wrap correctly. Wait until your little one is in a better mood and have a 'dry run' with a doll or a teddy, even if this is a poor substitute for the real thing. It is hard to imagine where and how tiny baby feet can get caught all over the place, how little hands can get into closed shirt pockets, why the tight T–shirt suddenly has countless folds for all possible baby body parts to get caught in. For the initial attempts many mothers wish they were wearing a skin-tight wetsuit – perhaps a body suit would do the same job.

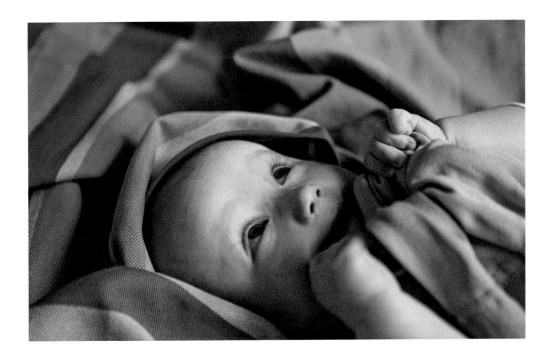

How to make life simpler

Wash, wash, wash! Stick your brand new wrap in the washing machine, use it as a voluminous shawl, sleep on it, pull and tug it around, in fact do everything to make sure it is no longer new and feels flexible and soft. A new wrap, with its bright colours, makes tying quite difficult. If it is stiff, it does not grip the baby and it is more difficult to tighten the knot. Maybe you could borrow a used wrap from a friend to practice with the first few times. You can tell at a distance whether a wrap is new or well-worn.

Choice of colour

With regard to the choice of colour, this is usually a matter of personal taste. Nowadays there are beguiling patterns and colour shades, the imagination of the manufacturers knows no limits and you can revel

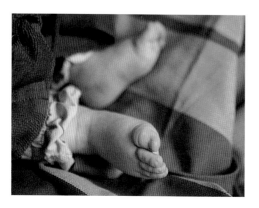

enthusiastically in the range of colours. However, as a wrap-tying novice, you may want to consider whether you could make your life a little easier by compromising here. With the different tying techniques, some of the material folds often need to be tightened. If the wrap has stripes lengthways, you will find it easier to recognise the loose section, even if you have inadvertently twisted it over to the back – this is particularly true if the stripes are arranged asymmetrically. Of course, distinguishable threads that stretch the length of the material can also help until you are confident enough in handling this material monster so that you don't have to completely give up your colour requirements.

Marking the centre

With most tying techniques, the centre of the material is the guide for the length distribution of the material. Manufacturers usually mark this point with a small woven mark, sewn on label or similar. For a beginner, however, it is practical if the marking runs across the whole piece of material, as it often bundles up or you turn up the edges at the start of tying and the label disappears between the folds. You can also just use a needle and thread to mark the centre.

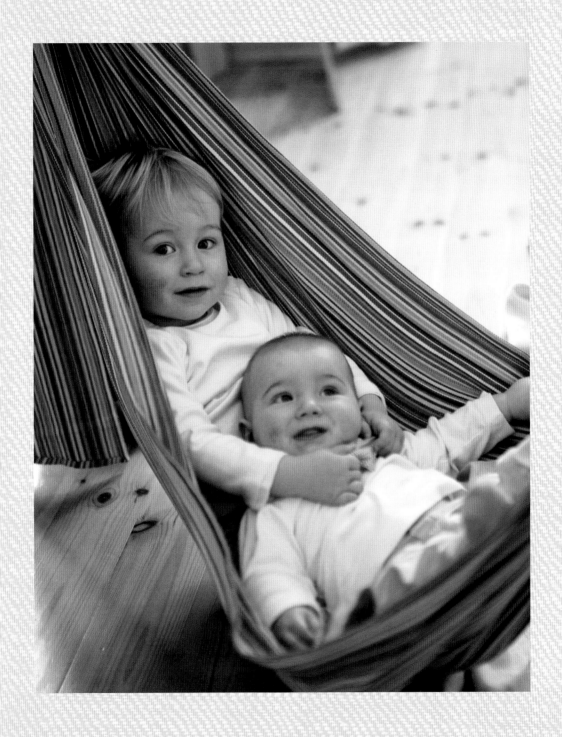

The knots

The different tying techniques usually end with a double knot, but it can't be just any knot. The familiar reef knot is recommended here. When you have wound the two material ends past each other, you need to stuff the right end of the material through the 'eyelet' you've formed from above. This is the trick. End 1 ultimately forms a complete loop running downwards, while end 2 forms one running upwards.

The advantage of this knot is that it lies flat and does not press on you and it is also easy to loosen if you have to tighten several folds of the material again at the end. A different double knot would tighten as soon as the weight of the child pulls on the material, whereby the material becomes looser and the knot is tightened into a round, fat lump. This then presses on your back and is hard to loosen.

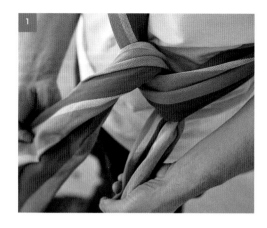

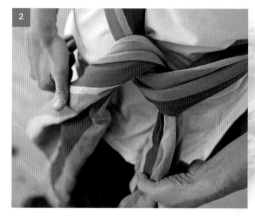

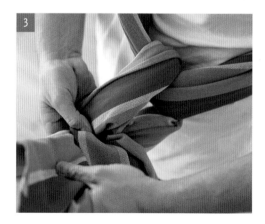

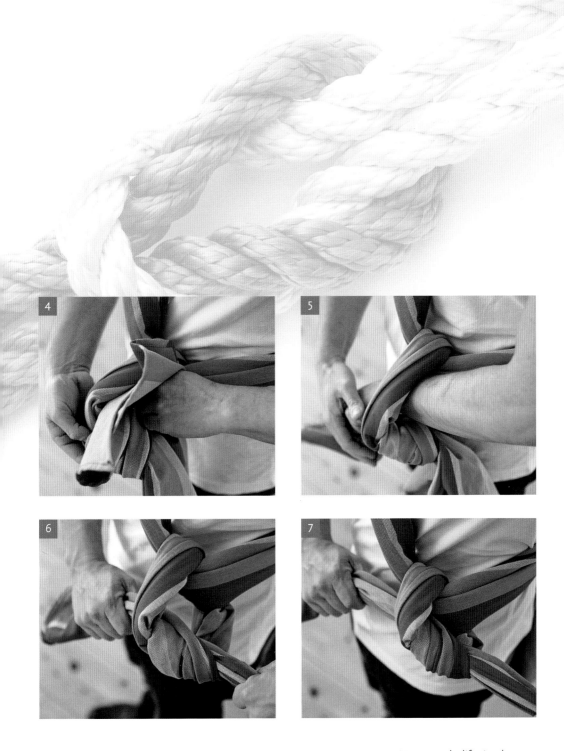

The material length and width

Experience shows that material with a width of around 70cm (27in) has proved to be the best. Only wraps for premature babies, stretchy or not, and very small, delicate babies are narrower (for more on stretchy wraps, see page 132). The answer isn't quite so simple for the material length, as you need a different minimum length depending on the tying-variation that you choose. The required sizes are given for each variant for an average body size (UK dress size 10–12, US 8–10). The wrap manufacturers provide lists from which you can determine the correct length for your body size and specific tying method. So before you make your purchase, you need to have some idea of how you want to carry your baby. If in doubt, go for a longer wrap. Otherwise, you will be a little annoyed when you can't use your selected tying technique, just because your material is a few centimetres short. Lengthening it isn't really an option. Midwives and babywearing educators, as well as parenting centres, also often function as 'wrap exchanges'; if you have made the wrong choice, there is certainly a solution. A survey of parents also showed that nowadays they often own several different wraps and carrying systems. Outgrown wraps can also be recycled as voluminous winter shawls and small hammocks, or remodelled as Mei Tai carriers.

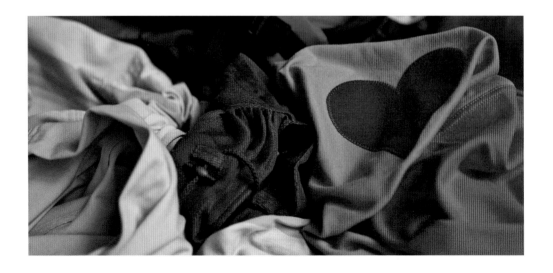

The quality of wraps

Of course you can also make your own wrap. African women use ordinary woven fabric. Just remember that the tying techniques used in Africa do not suit the majority of Europeans. Often two pieces of fabric are tied on top of one another, which is hard to identify in conventional images. In addition, Africans constantly retie when something becomes loose. This happens in an amazingly automatic way. For us in the West, this would be more than distracting, particularly in the colder seasons. With the tying techniques commonly used here, additional requirements are placed on the material.

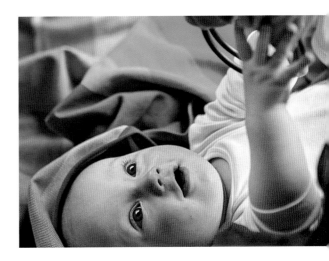

Stable in both the horizontal and vertical directions

The material must not yield in either the vertical or horizontal direction – in other words, in warp and weft – otherwise, if your child stays in the wrap for a long time, it will soon lose its shape.

Elastic on the diagonal

This means that the fabric yields in the diagonal direction but returns to shape when pressure is released. This ability to yield diagonally and return to shape is one of the factors that differentiates a wrap made from good material from a wrap of average quality. A baby must be closely held so that his upright body position is sufficiently stabilised. After the initial handholds and tying, each loose fold must be tightened so that the wrap is tight all over against the body of the child. If the material is too stiff and unyielding, this will not be particularly successful and will be hard work and rather tedious. When one fold is too loose, another is knotted up. If your baby moves, all your efforts were in vain as the stiff material no longer hugs your baby evenly. The knot is also difficult to tighten. If the material becomes stretched, the movement of your child also takes the whole thing out of shape. One part of the material lies flat; in another the fold is too loose. Just as in the case of more yielding warp and weft, you must retie and tighten the folds.

What sets a good wrap apart from others

- *An extensive weaving technique.* A simple fabric cannot meet the required strength and elasticity – particularly in the diagonal direction. A thin, simply woven material may cut in if the folds are pushed together. The danger exists in the neck and shoulder areas of the child and, in particular, in the hollow of the knees so that the legs can 'go to sleep'. I don't even want to talk about the effect on the parent's shoulders! On the other hand, a material that is too thick is difficult to handle.
- *A suitable surface structure and twist of fibres.* The warp threads and the weft are different. The material must not be too smooth, otherwise the knots gradually loosen. A structure that is too rough makes it more difficult to tighten the knot and the material folds are hard to tighten as the threads don't slide against each other easily. Apart from that, normal baby clothing sticks to the material too much when your child is sliding into a tied wrap. This makes the process unnecessarily slow and soon puts the baby in a bad mood.

- *Two-layered material edges.* The edges should be hemmed twice as the normal woven selvages soon give way, wear out and become warped.
- *Bevelled wrap ends.* These are very practical.

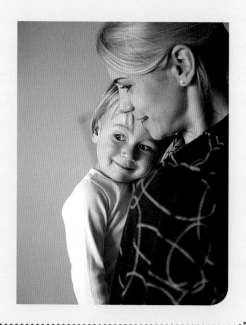

There are even differences between good, well-woven wraps, which experienced wrap users can explain. The consumer test journals I've mentioned also examine and judge new products. Obviously the fabric of a good wrap will loosen somewhat over time, but not enough to require correction during one carrying session. Even if a tying method allows you to reuse a tied wrap over and over, it is irritating to lose this advantage because the material is unsuitable.

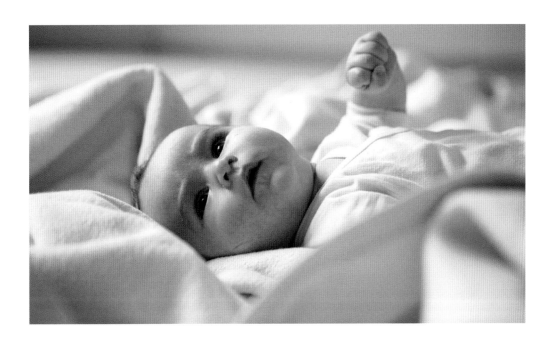

Addendum: stretchy wraps for little ones

Parents can easily bundle their baby in this type of wrap after first tying it in the appropriate way, as the elasticity means the wrap can be stretched in order to put the baby inside. His position is then easy to check and can be easily corrected because the elastic material can stretch slightly and will hug the baby tightly again immediately. For some parents, the stretchy wrap is *the* alternative for very sensitive, delicate and premature babies – even if you can use non-elastic wraps just as well in most cases with just a little bit of skill. To guarantee sufficient support, a 'three-layer' tying technique is important. The wrap cross carry (waist sash 'inside' and 'outside') has also proved to be particularly good in this case as it is suitable for very small babies and when the parents are initially inexperienced at tying. The baby can then be easily taken in and out of the wrap and the material still hugs the baby close.

However, the tying of these stretchy wraps requires particular care to ensure that the body position of the little one is sufficiently and correctly supported. In comparison to the 'normal' wraps, it must be tied really tightly so that the baby is held securely. Novice parents should be instructed in the correct handling by a competent person and, after trying them both out, they can then decide whether a stretchy or a normal woven wrap is more suitable for them.

More and more stretchy wraps have come onto the market. Not all meet the quality requirement that they should be both stretchy and, at the same time, strong enough to stabilise the position of the child. Sometimes the really stretchy synthetic elastic known as Lycra forms part of the material. (In America this is known as Spandex.) This artificial fibre content can be particularly unpleasant on hot days, but on the other hand delicate children can cool down quicker with this material than with stretchy wraps made of pure cotton. Take advice from experienced users.

Because of their characteristics, stretchy wraps are made specifically for premature babies or newborns and are thus somewhat smaller than normal woven wraps, which are recommended by manufacturers for a child weighing up to nine or ten kilograms (22 or 22lbs). Opinions differ on this matter and for many babywearers used to the normal' wraps, a stretchy wrap is too elastic even at significantly lower weights and does not support the baby sufficiently. **In any case, with a baby weighing upwards of about 6 kg, you should constantly check whether the wrap is still offering as much support as before and consider**

whether a different wrap might be more suitable. As soon as you feel that your baby can pull the stretchy wrap out of shape, you should switch to the normal woven variety, even if you have to do without some of the practical aspects of the stretchy wrap.

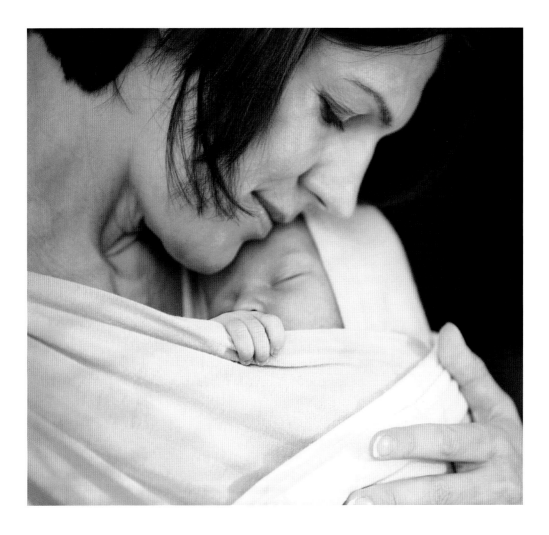

Different tying techniques

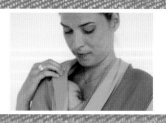

General information for the different techniques

The following tying techniques have some basic points in common, which you should heed when tying and which should facilitate both tying and carrying.

Preparation and folding the edge

To make the material easier to use before tying, you can spread it out centred across your arm and pull it together with small equal folds. Or – particularly for very small newborn and premature babies – you can make the material narrower by folding it over lengthways along both sides. When tying, these turned over sections of material lie to the *outside*. The term 'folded edge' then refers to the edge that was created by folding, not the actual edge of the material. The material is thus doubled and provides good support in the area of the child's shoulders and back. If

you want to support the child's head, you can pull this folded section upwards and open it up.

Tightening the folds

This I have already mentioned earlier, but, as it is an important point, I would like to look at it again in more detail. For good support, the sections of material must closely hug your baby. This rarely happens on the first attempt. As soon as your child is sitting in the wrap, the sections of material that are too loose must be tightened fold for fold or – as it is often described – strand by strand and from the middle of the child's back to the right *and* left, so that he is not tilted to one side. Therefore it can be useful if you do not pull the knot tight at the start and wait until the loose folds have been included evenly in the knot before tightening.

Distribution of weight

You should carry your child tied up high in the wrap because the weight distribution is better for you as the babywearer. The lower the centre of gravity, the harder it is to carry the baby. On the other hand, there should be no risk of you inadvertently knocking the delicate baby fontanelles with your chin. You may have heard the phrase 'Close enough to kiss' in relation to babywearing, which means that if you tip your head forward you should be able to kiss your baby on the head (This is one of the 'T.I.C.K.S.' rules for safe babywearing you can find on the internet.) Of course, you should avoid having his head within your field of vision as much as possible, as it is easy to stumble when you can't see the next step. You should take great care when climbing stairs.

'Pulling downwards' or 'crossing' the material over the shoulders

If you want to pull the section of material along the head or the child's shoulders even tighter to better support them, pull the wrap down off your shoulders. To do this, you can either simply pull the edge of the material by your neck down over the shoulders from above (see Fig. page 149, right), or, you can pull this neck edge 'down and through'. In other words, grasp through under the material on your shoulder and grasp the edge which is also going to the back of your child. Now pull this material edge down and through the material (which is also going to sit in the baby's knee hollows) and downwards over the shoulder (see Fig. page 143). This 'pulling down' also prevents the wrap from pressing on the area near your neck. In doing this, however, you will find that the freedom of movement in your arms is somewhat restricted.

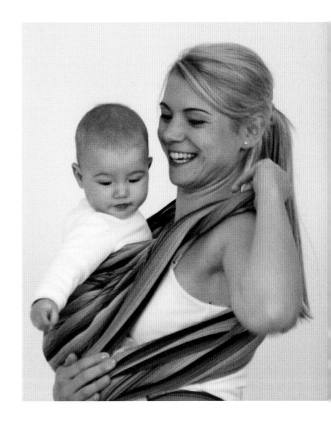

Sitting upright on the chest 1: The classic 'Wrap Cross Carry' or 'Front Wrap Cross Carry' (FWCC)

Material length
Approx. 4.75m (15 1/2 ft) and longer.

What you need to know
- Suitable from early on and particularly good for little ones.
- The wrap is usually retied each time, but the child can also be taken out and put back in, particularly with the variant 'waist sash outside'.

Note
Particularly good for very little babies as even novice parents can get on with this and so the baby is more likely to be in the correct position.

Preparation
- Mark the middle of the material.
- If necessary, fold over the material lengthways on both sides, particularly for very small babies.

How to do it
1. Wrap the material around your waist like a high sash. The centre of the material should be at the centre of your body (any folded over edges are on the outside) – it doesn't matter if the upper edge reaches your armpits.
2. Pass one end of the material after the other across your back and then up and over your shoulders to the front, so that the material crosses on your back. Make sure that the

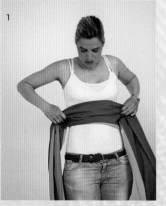
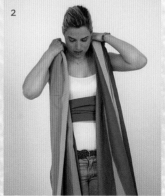
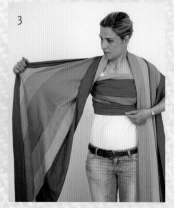

sections of material are not twisted – this makes it easier to tighten the material folds. First tighten the material section lying underneath on your back and then the upper section – the waist sash should now be tight.

3 Check the folded edges again and, if necessary, pull to tighten – in particular tighten the folds that will later lie in the backs of your child's knees (lower edge of your waist sash) and those that will later hug his head and shoulders (upper edge of your waist sash).

The folds that sit in the backs of the knees must be pulled tight so the child is in the tucked leg position. The material can be pulled so tight that it almost seems impossible that a baby could fit in there. If the material is already pulled close, it takes less effort to tighten it with the child inside.

What's next: it isn't as difficult as it may seem when reading or when trying it out for the first time. Once you have managed it and your baby is settled as before, then:

4 Lay your baby over a shoulder and let him slowly slide into the waist sash, initially with moderately stretched legs.

As soon as possible, try to spread his legs and tuck them up a little bit. To do this you will probably have to reach into the material with your hand from below to achieve the spread and squat position. Take your time to sort out the legs; his feet can get caught in all sorts of places!

5 As soon as his legs are in the spread–squat position and the lower legs are outside of the wrap, you have almost made it. If your material is pulled tight from the start, you can assume that it is also holding your child securely, even though the material is not yet

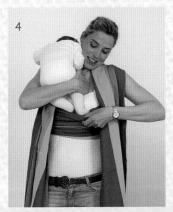
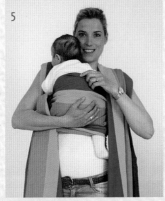
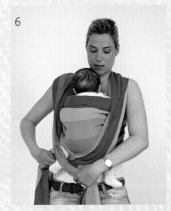

knotted. You can now carry on in peace. Tighten the material fold by fold again over the child as necessary. When doing this you can also pull the material that was folded over at the start over the head to give your baby support if he is still small. When you are sure that your child is tightly packed and is in the correct position, you can proceed at your leisure.

6 Pull the sections of material down, cross them under the baby's bottom and pull them under his legs through to your back. Tie the knot on your back. The material sections in the hollow of the baby's knees supports the tuck bosition of the legs.

Finally, pull apart the lower section of material from the hollow of one knee to the other and spread it out across your baby's back, then do the same for the upper section of material.

Variant for a shorter piece of material

Do not pull out the parts of material over the baby's back. Instead, pull them down to the right and left of his body and make the knot under his bottom, not on your back. In this case the legs really should be well-squatted from the start. The knot can, however, slip upwards so you should regularly check it.

Variant 'Waist Sash Outside' or 'Pocket Wrap Cross Carry (PWCC)

From 'What's next' on page 137, stuff the two hanging material ends into the waist sash and pull them down. The material ends are now inside and the waist sash is outside on top. Then cross over the material ends under the sash and under the baby's bottom. Finally pull them through under his legs and knot them at your back. This variant is almost identical to the classic 'waist sash inside' described in detail above, but it requires more practice as it is harder to pull the material tight. The 'outside' variant is often used for stretchy wraps.

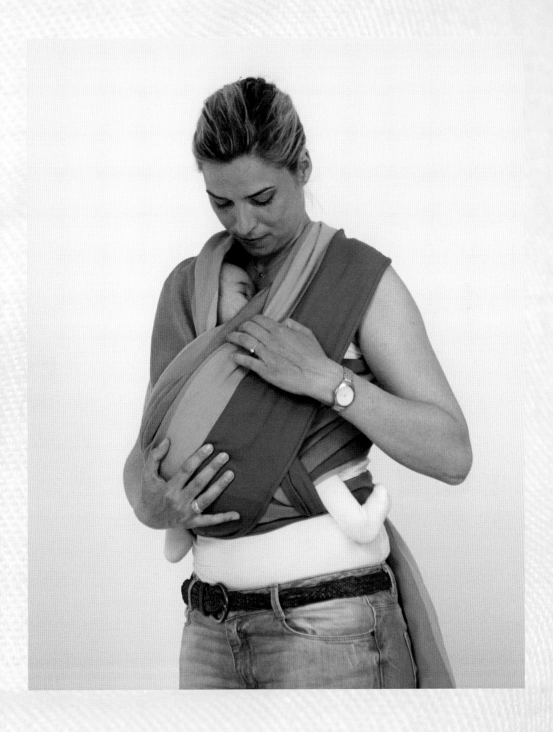

Sitting upright on the chest 2:
The 'Kangaroo Sling' or 'Kangaroo Carry'

Material length
Approx. 3.75m (12 1/4ft) and longer

What you need to know
- Experienced wrap users can achieve a correct position immediately, even with very small babies.
- The wrap is retied each time.

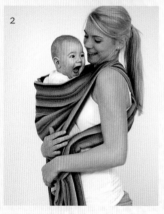

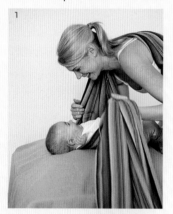

Note
This variation of tying is hard for new wrap users, particularly with new material and newborns!

Preparation
- Mark the middle of the material.
- Spread out the material on a table.
- If necessary, fold over the material lengthways along one or both sides.

How to do it
1 Place your baby at the mid-point of the material. Important: for very small babies, place the head completely on the material. Bend over your baby and place the ends of the material over your shoulders – it is best to arrange them in a cross on your back at this point as your hands are free. After this you can lay the ends over your lower arms.
2 Gather up some material in the backs of your baby's knees. Lift up your child with the material and in a secure hold. Pull the material ends lying diagonally over your back through under your arms to the front if you didn't before – the material must not be twisted and should be flat against your back and spread out.

   Tighten the sections of material – first the

lower one – in particular the folds in the backs of your baby's knees which support the correct tucked position.

Check the folds in the spinal area and, if necessary, tighten them again. Cross the ends of the material under the baby's bottom.

4 Pull each of them backwards under the legs. Tie the knot at your back. Check the tucked position of the legs. If necessary, pull the material down over your shoulders (see p135).

Variant for a shorter piece of material
If you have a shorter piece of material, you can end this tying method with a reef knot under the child's bottom.

Note
This tying method may sound easier than the wrap cross carry. However, tightening the folds so that your baby's back is supported correctly is difficult, particularly in the first weeks of life. Your baby is still very small and you are a wrap novice who must tighten the material while securely supporting the baby.

There are other variations to this technique. For example, some people roll together the sections of material over the shoulders of the carrying person like a cord. However, in this case you can no longer tighten the material folds. The child's leg position and the support of his back must therefore be correct and adequate from the start.

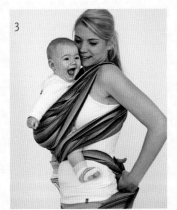

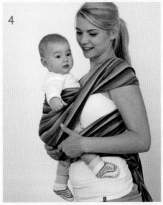

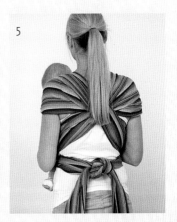

Feet in or feet out?

The wrap cross carry and kangaroo tying methods can be adapted so that the material covers the feet. As usual, there are different methods for this. The sections of material crossed under the baby's bottom can be tied in a special way so that the feet are 'included' and supported. Alternatively, the material which otherwise reaches to the backs of the knees can be pulled down until the lower legs and feet are completely enclosed by the material. However, this is mostly at the expense of a well-supported tucked position.

Some newborns are calmer if their feet are enclosed. For these babies you can try exerting pressure on the soles of the feet to offset digestive problems, as in kinesiology, but for this you will need an introduction to tying techniques from an expert. To pack the feet into the material and still maintain a tuck position of 100° or 110° is difficult and needs expert advice.

Some websites suggest that enclosing the feet is essential for the first four months. There are no sound arguments for this rule. In addition, with these types of carrying techniques, the feet may be fixed in a particular position for hours at a time, which could cause malformations. And, as already mentioned, the tucked position is often not achieved. If the material only reaches to the backs of the knees, you are giving your baby more chance to move freely, which is generally seen as positive for motor development.

Older children may push down on the material with their feet and push themselves up, which can pull the whole wrap out of shape.

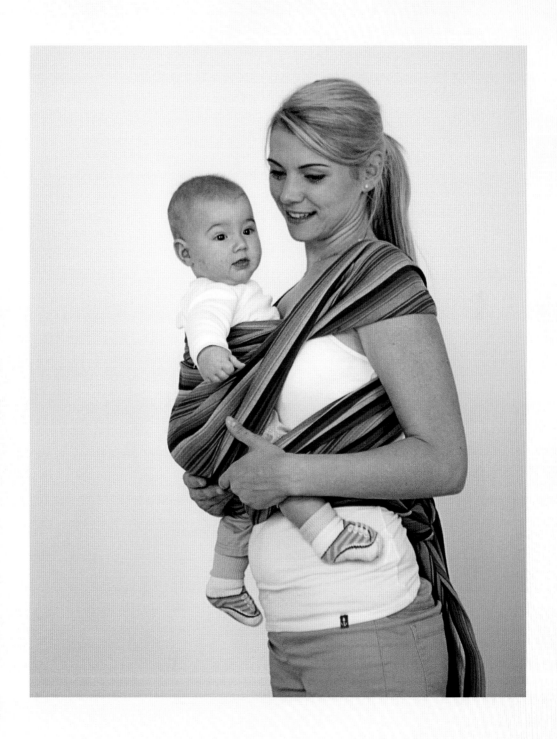

Sitting upright on the chest 3:
The classic 'Cross Carry' or 'Front Cross Carry' (FCC)

Material length
From approx. 4.25m (3 1/2ft)

What you need to know
- For babies who are more stable in the spine, so from approximately two to three months.
- The wrap can remain tied when the baby is taken out.

Note
Less suitable for the first weeks of life when babies fall easily to the side. If used correctly, the cross carry is a very easy variant, and a child can be quickly taken out of the wrap and put in, without the need to re-tie.

Preparation
- Form a loop a good two hands wide near the centre of the material.

How to do it
1 Swing the loop over your head and position it on your back above your waist. The ends with unequal length hang down in front from the shoulders – one half of the material can be 20 to 30cm (8 to 12in) longer. In this way, you can tie the knot at the side, which is easier than tying it to the back.
2 Pull the longer end across your front and through under your arm to your back and through the loop at your back.
3 Then pull this long end back through to the front under the other arm.

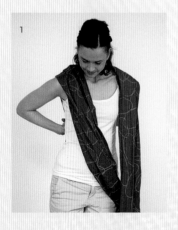
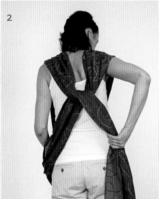
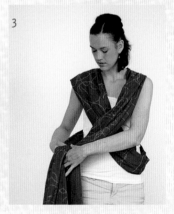

4 Knot the two ends of the material to the side at hip height – slightly towards your back so that the knot doesn't hurt your baby. The sections of material now form a cross in front of your chest. Push this material cross downwards a little bit.

5 Now lay your baby over one shoulder and let the legs slowly slide into the upper V-section of the wrap. The legs must be directed out to the side one after the other under the material sections so that your baby ultimately sits on the cross of material.

6 Hold your baby with one arm and first expand the section of material next to the body across the nappy from the hollow of one knee to the other, then do the same with the external section of material. Next help him to achieve the tuck position.

Note
With agile children, make sure that they do not squash the sections of material between their legs. By expanding the sections of material from the hollow of one knee to the other, you also expand the material broadly across the back of the child. With older children, the shoulders may peep out of the upper V, but not too wide, otherwise the back may not be correctly supported.

Now you can decide

• . . . whether your child's arms stay in the wrap and his head is also supported by the fabric if he is asleep,

• or whether – if he's a little, lively and stable sitting baby – his arms should be free so that he can be more proactive.

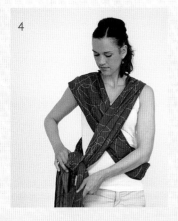

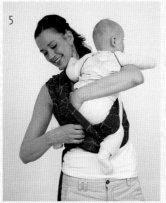

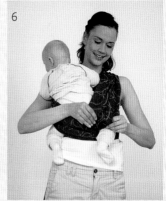

The 'rounded back position'

The overall rounded appearance of the child's back during infancy is the result of the immature lumbar lordosis and the lack of a distinct cervical lordosis (see page 35). The latter develops as soon as an infant begins to lift his head. The lumbar lordosis, which is initially slight, increases gradually as soon as a child sits upright, begins to crawl and walk and takes more exercise. However, when carrying a baby, he should not be forced into a strongly rounded position, particularly in the cervical (neck) vertebrae. Instead he should have the option to be upright in the shoulder area and lift his head, as the cervical lordosis is encouraged by use. When being carried, he should be able to look independently into the parent's face. This trains the appropriate muscles as it stimulates the baby to lift his head and thus encourages the development of the cervical lordosis and head control. Having an extremely rounded position, particularly after the new-born stage, removes the chance for a baby to use this little training programme. Parents automatically provide the correct level of rounding in the spinal area when they create a good tucked position, and the baby can lean on their body and sit upright in this way. It will probably be more of a stretched incomplete C than a semi-circular round. This encouragement of cervical lordosis has become important today as, to prevent sudden infant death syndrome (SIDS), babies spend the majority of their day lying on their backs. They are missing the incentive to push up from lying on their stomachs to see the environment around them. As a result they are also missing out on a significant period of time when they can exercise their arm and neck muscles. Babies who sleep on their backs take longer to turn over, sit, crawl and push themselves up.[97]

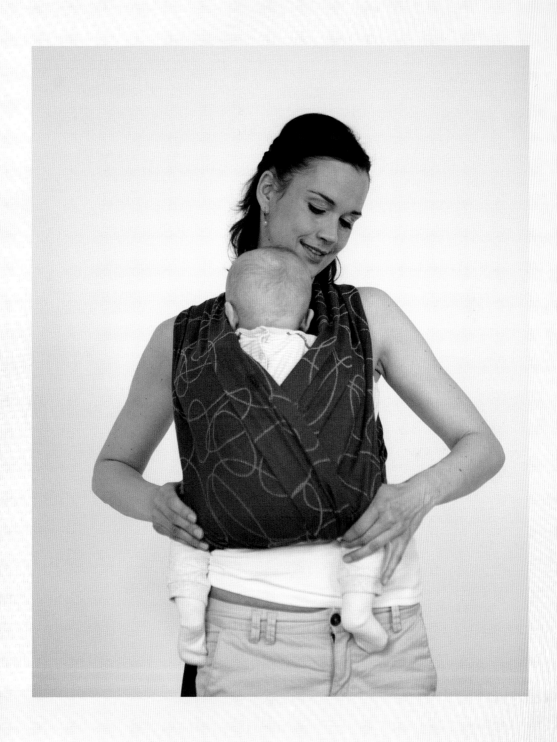

Upright to the side on the hip 1:
The classic 'Lateral Hip Carry' or 'Simple Hip Carry'

Material length
Approx. 2.75m (9ft) – a bit longer is better

What you need to know
- Suitable for curious, restless little people who want to see more of the world, but also suitable for very small babies.

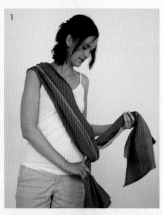

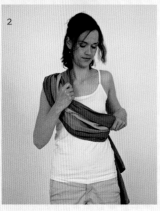

- When the wrap is tied correctly once, it can be used in the same way in the future.
- The hip carry is particularly good for the healthy development of the infantile hip joints (see page 48).

Preparation
- Mark the middle of the material.
- Find and mark the top and bottom edges of the material (important if you later want to use the tied wrap again correctly).
- For very small babies, fold over the material lengthways to reduce the width.

How to do it the first time
1. Place the centre of the material on the right shoulder – the baby will be sitting on the left hip. The parent has the right hand free. (Most people are right-handed – strangely enough, left-handed people automatically carry their babies on their left hip too unless they have to carry something by hand).
2. Tie the material with a flat reef knot at hip height on the left but do not pull it tight – the material should be lying diagonally across your upper body. With very small babies, plan a smaller loop. Then push the knot between the shoulder blades.

3 Let your baby slide down into the wrap from the shoulder – at the start you may feel safer if you place your left foot somewhere raised. Your child can then find support on your thigh. With larger and heavier children, this is also a good way to reduce the weight until the wrap is sorted out. When sliding the baby into the wrap, the legs should come into the spread–squat position.

4 When your baby is sitting on your hip, check the leg position again – the material can easily form a thick bulge at the hollows/backs of the knees, and it will not constrict there. Important: the legs of the child must be well bent up, otherwise you may feel that your baby could slide out – a sure sign that he is not sitting correctly in the wrap. If necessary support the body position of your child while someone loosens the knot at your back so that the loose sections of material can be tightened – take your time over this, as the thorough tightening of the folds guarantees your baby's correct position. When your baby is securely positioned, tighten the knot. If the material in your child's shoulder and head area is double–layered, it is easier to pull the material over the head.

5 If you pull down the edge of the material by your neck (the edge in your child's head–back area) over your shoulder, the material will hug your baby closer in the head–shoulder area.

Variant for very small babies

Very small babies can be laid on the wrap already tied as a loop. If you then slip an arm into the loop in which your baby is already lying and pull the material over your head, you can safely support your baby. Mark on the wrap where you must correctly position your baby so that next time you can immediately find the correct place him in the loop.

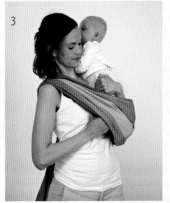
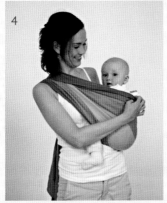
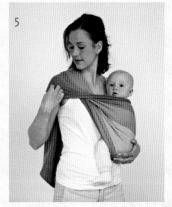

Variant 1 for older babies

- Tie the loop as described above or arrange the tied wrap according to upper and lower edge.
- Position the knot to the front on your chest, approximately at the height of your armpit (the knot is moved forward and is not on your back, thus it is easy to access).
- Place your foot on a chair.
- Slide your child into the wrap from above until he is sitting on your thigh in the wrap.

Variant 2 for older babies

- Place your baby on your thigh.
- Bundle up the lower half of the material (the knot is at the front)
- Pull the material over your child's back to the hollows of the knees when the legs are in a tucked position. When doing this, fan out the bundle of material gradually.
- As the knot is to the front, you can, if necessary, tighten individual folds yourself. You can, of course, position the knot to your back as for little babies if the material is already tied well.

Note

I admit that the lateral hip carry is my favourite wrap variant. Even small babies who cannot control their own head are able to decide for themselves if they want to 'see something of the world', make eye contact with mummy or daddy or turn their face towards the person carrying them if the stimulation becomes too much. Babies can thus decide by themselves whether to turn towards the world, or not, in accordance with their mood. Unfortunately, this method may not be easy on the mother's back, particularly if this is already a problem area, because the person carrying invariably adopts a slightly tilted posture as soon as a baby sits on the hip, with or without a wrap.

(But may I remind you again here of the preventative effect on hip dysplasia due to the spread–squat position (see page 48) and also the fact that the circulation is improved in the baby's hip joint area when in a lateral hip carry.)

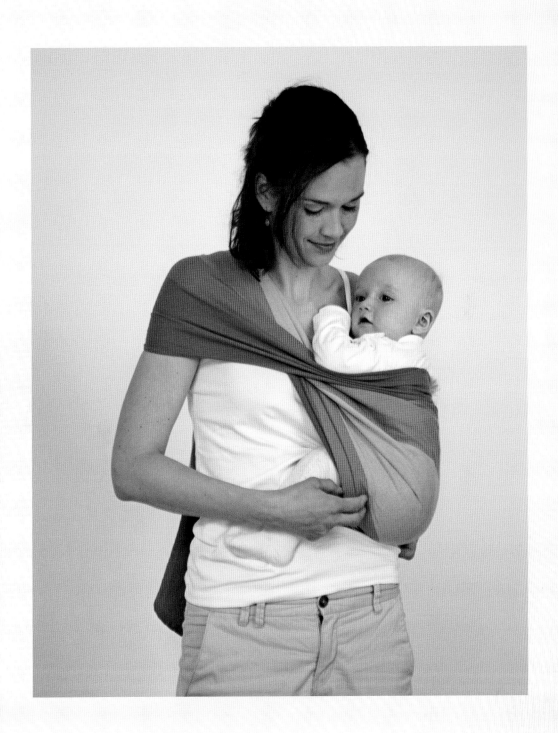

Upright to the side on the hip 2:
The 'Hip Sling' or the 'Robin's/Poppins Hip Carry'

Material length

Approx. 3.75m (12 1/4ft) – and longer for older babies

What you need to know

- Suitable for curious, restless little people.
- The material sections that are too loose are somewhat harder to tighten than with the 'side hip carry', so this is better for older babies.
- The material must be re-tied for each carrying period, but you can take your child in and out several times within each period without re-tying.
- While a short piece of material is better for the 'classic hip carry' (if the ends are too long, it can be annoying), this lateral carrying variant requires a longer piece of mate-rial.
- Again, this is particularly good for the development of the infantile hip joints (see page 48).

Preparation

1 Lay the material over your shoulder so that the centre is on your shoulder. End 1 is to the front, end 2 lies to the back.

How to do it

2 With the left hand, reach behind and pull the rear end of the material (no. 2) under your left armpit through to the front, straight across your chest and over the other end at the front (no. 1).

3 Throw the front end hanging down (no. 1) over your shoulder to the back so that the material forms a loop on your chest and the other end of the wrap (no. 2) is placed inside it.

4 Spread out the wrap on your shoulder – this distributes the weight of your child.

5 Reach behind with the left hand and bring the other end (no. 1) to the front.

6 Tie a single knot under the pouch (half reef knot).

7 Spread out the pouch for your child.

8 Slide the baby into the pouch from above. Check that the folds sit well; if necessary, pull loose folds of material through the loop. Twist the ends of the material into a full reef knot.

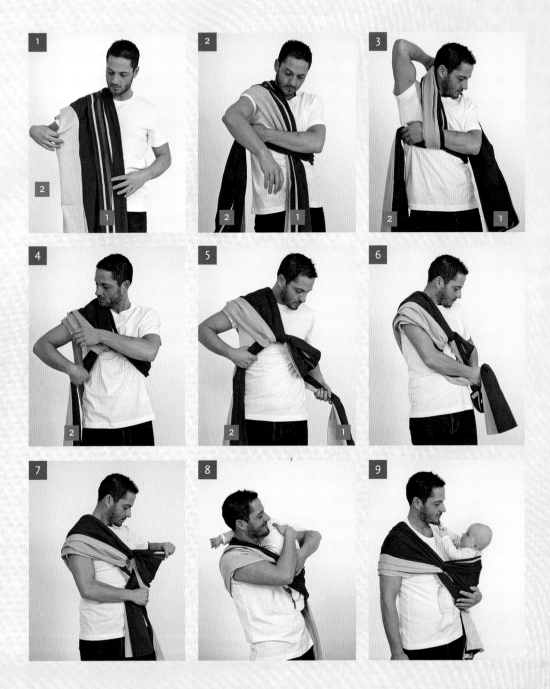

Upright to the side on the hip 2: The 'Hip Sling' or the 'Robin's/Poppins Hip Carry'   153

The variant for more practised parents:

- Fold the material over with one side two to three hand widths longer than the other.
- Reach into the loop and lay the folded material over the right shoulder from behind. Pull the loop down a little bit lower than the armpit. Both parts of the material are lying folded on your shoulder and hang down over your back. The longer section of material (no. 1) should be on the bottom.
- Reach behind with your left hand and pull the longer part (no. 1) under your left armpit to the front.
- Pull the end of the material through the loop from the left (see page 153, Fig. 4) – this creates the carrying pouch on the left hip.
- Continue from step 4 as described above.

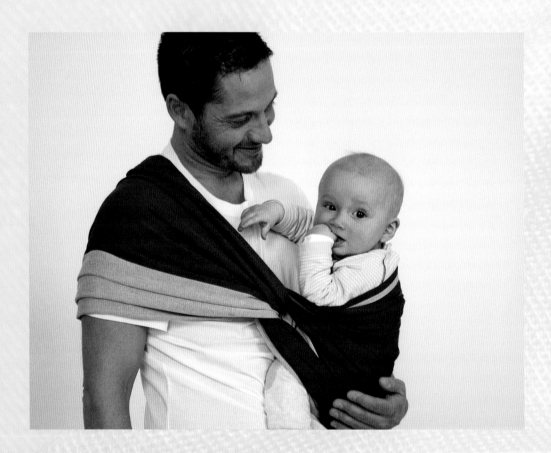

Carrying on your back: the 'Rucksack Wrap'

Material length
From approx. 3.75m (12 1/4ft)

What you need to know
- A tying variant for older children who can already control their head well and want to see more than they can when sitting to the front.
- Children of over two years can still be carried, as the tying method is similar to a close-fitting rucksack.
- Experienced wrap users can carry quite small babies on their backs to keep them out of danger when cooking or washing up. In this case, the head must also be securely supported. This means that the baby is sitting low enough so that the material also covers the head.
- The wrap must be re-tied each time.

Note
This tying method is not that different from the kangaroo sling. It is just more complicated, as your baby must be tied to your back out of your direct field of vision, and thus also out of direct reach. This makes you less confident.

Some people also tie their little ones in the 'reverse' wrap cross carry (also called back wrap across carry – BWCC), but for breastfeeding women in particular this can cause uncomfortable pressure as the material crosses over the chest. Experienced fathers obviously don't have a problem with this. Imaginative wrap users have found solutions but there is not space for them here; an internet search will help if you are interested.

The description for the simpler procedure for older babies is followed by further instructions on how the child can be placed on your back. These certainly give only an indication of the available options. Older babies who are used to the wrap can be placed on the back and the material spread over them. Little ones also remain calmly on your back if you bend down and they are used to this. But nothing's easy to start off with and you should get help from someone with experience. Don't be disheartened by images of African mothers for whom everything seems to work wonderfully and even the smallest baby lies huddled up on the back in absolute calm until it is tied in the wrap.

With regard to posture, the back carrying method is just as suitable for a child as a front carrying method provided that you pay attention to the same points – support the back and head and ensure a good tucked position.

Another note on the correct height for the baby: to best distribute the weight for the babywearer, the child should be tied as high as possible (see page 135). Older babies can then look over your shoulder, participate more and also communicate with you. Smaller babies must sit lower so that their head is supported by the material. Eye contact is then no longer possible. But little babies are usually carried on the back for short periods only, when the front method is not suitable at that particular moment.

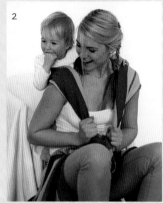

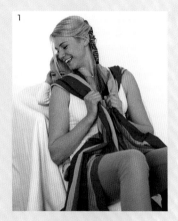

Preparation – variant for children with good head and body control

- Ideally spread out the material over an armchair (across the back and arms).
- Place your baby in the material and drape it once around the hollows of the knees.

How to do it

1 Pull the material under the child's armpits. Sit in front of your child and lean back slightly. Pull the ends of the material forwards over your shoulders – it is best to let them slide through the hands several times so that the material folds lie parallel – and hold both material sections in front of your chest.

2 Bend forward – your child is now on your back. Check that the legs are in a good tuck position. If necessary, pull the material tighter around the child's shoulders.

3 As you gradually stand upright, you can choose between two different variants:
Carrying method for women: pull the ends of the material backwards directly under your armpits like the shoulder straps of a rucksack.
Carrying method for men: cross the ends of the material over your chest and pull backwards under the arms.

4 Cross over the ends of the material under the nappy, under the hollows of the knees, and pull back to the front.

5 Tie at the front. If the material is shorter end with the reef knot immediately under the child's bottom.

Variant for very small babies

It is best to lay very small babies on the wrap spread out on a bed. You have to lean a long way back as you pull the ends of the material over your shoulders; however, this strengthens your stomach muscles. You must, of course, make sure that your baby's head is inside the material. Then continue with the procedure described above.

Variant for very small babies and very competent parents (also called 'santa-toss' or 'over the shoulder')

- Position your baby in the centre of the material, which has been folded along its length so it is narrower than normal – it should enclose the whole head and reach the hollows of the knees when the legs are tucked.
- Bunch up the ends of the material with your left hand, just above the baby's body so that he is lying as in a swing with a slightly rounded back. If your baby is unsettled, you can swing it gently and calm him.
- Lift the little bundle to the right shoulder and support it with your right hand and lower arm.
- Next use some momentum and support from the right arm and swing the bundle to the right shoulder – if your child has been tied up correctly like a bundle with well tucked legs, he should now be lying securely with his head and stomach on your shoulder.
- Now grasp one of the ends with each hand and let the bundle slide slowly downwards.
- In the meantime take your left arm over your head so that now the ends of the

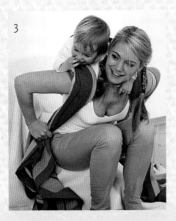

3

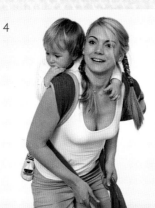

4

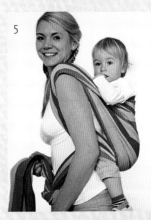

5

material are lying to the right and left over your shoulders.

- As soon as your child is at the correct height, continue as described above – you've finished. (You will probably be finished, too, when you first try this variant!)

Variant for smaller and lighter babies (also called 'hip-scoot')

- Put the material around your baby's shoulders.
- Place your child on one hand, with his back and head huddled into your lower arm and elbow.
- Push him backwards around your waist to the middle of your back – as high as possible on your body – while the other hand provides additional support for him. In the meantime bend forwards, still holding your baby with one hand.
- Arrange the material – then proceed as described above.

Elegant variant for babies who already have good head control (this is a variation of 'superman-toss')

I only want to introduce you to one more of the many variants. Try them out and see which one suits you best.

- Lay or place your child in the centre of the material, which should be spread out on the floor in front of you.
- Kneel behind him.

- Bend over your child (the upper edge of the material should be above his shoulders) and sit him slightly upright.
- Grasp your child together with the material edge from above/front under the armpits (thumbs gripping under the armpits, palms of the hand on your baby's chest. The handling is momentarily rather awkward).
- Lift your child and the material backwards over your head – the equal length ends of the material should now be hanging to the right and left over your shoulders.
- Bend forwards and lay down your baby on your back – he is now placed high up on your back.
- Grasp both ends of the material and let your child slide down to the correct height – tighten the folds and check the tuck position.

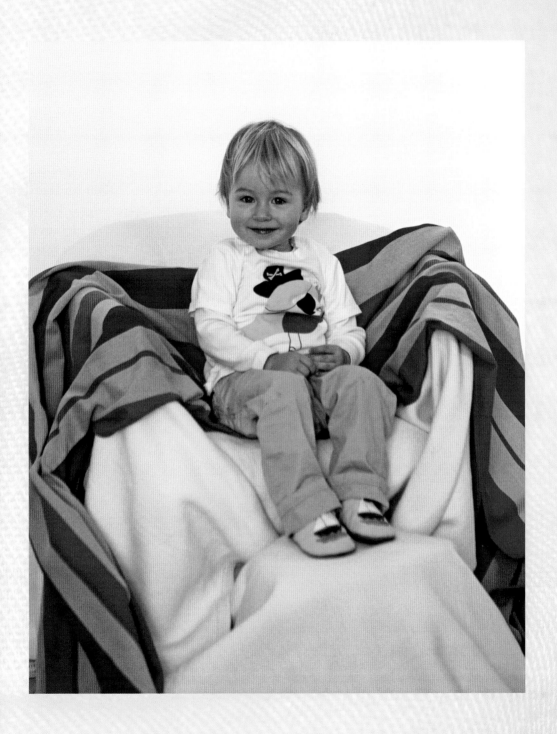

Carrying in a lying position: the 'Cradle Carry'

Material length

Approx. 2.75m (9ft) – ideally longer

What you need to know

- Only suitable for the first weeks of life.
- Once tied, the wrap is always ready to use.

Note

Some parents are reluctant to sit their newborn upright in a wrap and they prefer to carry their baby in a lying position for the first weeks of life. This is the only reason to choose a cradle carry method. However, the cradle is really only intended for very small babies. You lose the benefit of the spread–squat position, which prevents dysplasia if used early, as the legs are only slightly bent and not in a good tuck position. As soon as the head and/or the feet stick out past your body your baby has outgrown this position because there is a risk that he could be bumped in a moment of carelessness. In addition, with the cradle carry method, an older child is more bent up in the wrap and the chin is pressed onto the chest. This obstructs breathing. Your child also lies slightly to the side in the wrap. Make sure that he does not gradually turn towards you, following the natural curvature of his body, so that his face falls into the folds of the material.

If your baby prefers a lateral curved posture to one side, you should not encourage it with this tying method. This type of carrying can, however, be used to compensate slightly for this, if your baby tolerates it. If he is not carried on his 'best side', the little awkward customer will sometimes react in an extremely ungracious manner. But I don't mean that you can self-treat bad posture in a child in this way – that is a matter for a doctor. It seems that babies with conditions of this type are particularly difficult to carry in a lying position, so most parents then decide to use an upright carrying position, in which the baby often loses the tilted posture.

There are several methods of tying. I will present those in which the baby lies relatively straight, the face remains free and you can observe him, even when this is at the expense of good weight distribution. But this is not an issue as your little pipsqueak is still a lightweight!

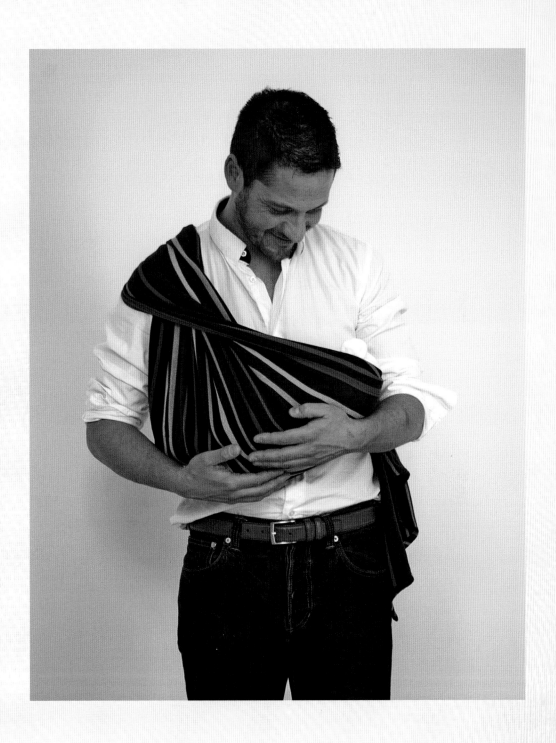

Preparation

1 With this variant, the child's head is orientated towards the arm, where the material runs under your shoulder to the back.

- Lay the wrap over the right or the left shoulder.
- Tie the ends of the material at the height of the left hip with a reef knot.
- Slip out of the wrap and spread the loop out on a table.

How to do it

2 Lay your baby near the centre of the material, (approximately one or two hand widths away), so that the head is completely covered by the material – in this way, the knot of the loop is placed on your spine so it does not cause uncomfortable pressure.

3 Slip your head and left arm – the baby's head is lying in this direction – into the wrap.

4 Slowly stand up with your child, support his body and arrange his head and upper body to the left. Important: always make sure that the baby's head is fully enclosed and supported.

5 When you are upright, position the knot exactly between your shoulder blades. With a bit of practice you will know how your baby should be positioned in the wrap from the start – so that you rarely have to adjust him.

6 Now you can pull down the material edge at your neck over your shoulder – this section of material is thus tightened around the head and shoulders of your baby and gently lifts them. In addition, the material doesn't

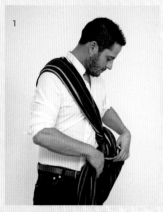

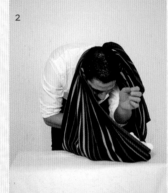

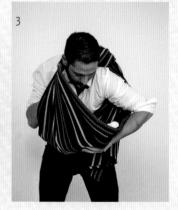

press so much in the neck area and the weight is distributed evenly across your shoulders.

If you have tied the wrap for the first time, you should check its position. To examine and correct the position of the wrap, however, someone must be available to tighten the folds and sort out the knot on your back.

Note

If you use the wrap again, you must mark which edge of the material is by your baby's head and which is by his feet so that the position is also correct the next time you use it.

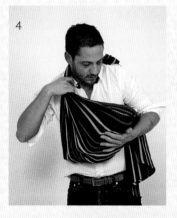
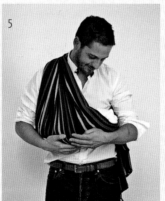
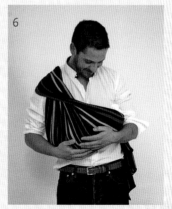

Wrap-like carriers: ring slings, pouches, Mei Tais, onbuhimos…

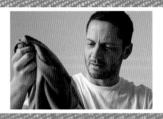

There are numerous carriers that are based on a wrap and often manufactured from wrap material. They are intended to be easier to use, with straps, rings or buckles. As a result of internet shopping in particular, the market has become more confusing and it is easy to buy unsuitable products. At the risk of sounding like a broken record, the following still applies: make sure you do your research.

Special features

- Quick to position baby in.
- As the baby can huddle in close to the person carrying him, the weight distribution is good for the person carrying.

Points to consider

- Some of these carriers can be used in a number of different ways, but not all of them can be adjusted to provide sufficient back support for babies of all ages.
- The more that a carrier can be adjusted, the more difficult it is to use, although it will get easier with practice.

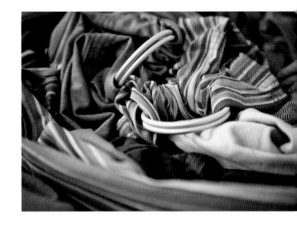

Ring slings

Special features
- *May* be suitable for all ages.
- A baby can be carried in all positions.

The ring sling more or less corresponds to a wrap tied in a lateral hip carry, in which a baby sits upright and can also be carried to the front or in the cradle position. The knot is replaced by a double ring system, which the material is drawn through to form the sitting pouch. With a suitable ring system and good quality material and manufacture, the material can be tightened fold by fold and adjusted to the child.

Some ring slings, however, are not suitable for small babies as the quality of the material, padding or reinforcements does not allow sufficient tightening of the folds in the back area. Some rings are too small, some rings loosen under weight, some materials lack the required elasticity. It is therefore important to try them out and research each product before buying.

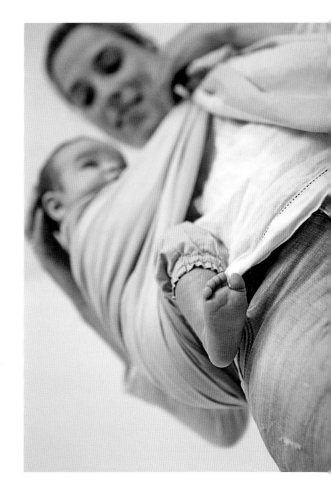

Pouches

Special features

- Quick to set up.

Bear in mind

- Limited adjustment options.
- The suggested carrying methods are often not recommended.

Another type of carrier is the pouch. In principle, a pouch is a hammock-like, wrap-like or sling-like product made completely of fabric and sometimes of stretchy material. They are not adjustable for everyday use, although some can be unpicked and re-sewn. Pouches enjoy great popularity in the USA and they are also available elsewhere through internet shopping. Products of this type must be considered with a critical eye, not least because they cannot be adjusted to suit the anatomy of each baby. Parents are encouraged to carry babies in a lying position. However, the little one is often too huddled up (see Fig. 11), and the chin is pushed onto the chest. This obstructs breathing, which can be critical for newborns or sick children, in particular.

Other pouches do not enclose a baby sufficiently and securely enough. If the parent then stumbles or the baby makes a strong movement, it can fall out. The result of these ill–thought-out designs is often a fractured skull, as accident statistics recorded in the USA show.[98] (See page 169.) The recommendation to push a baby in a pouch round to your back for carrying him, where he is completely out of reach, is very dangerous if the edges of the pouch are not tight and leave a wide gap.

As with ring slings, babies can also be carried upright in pouches. However, this is a prefabricated carrier, which can only be adjusted to the child's body and to the parents to a limited extent.

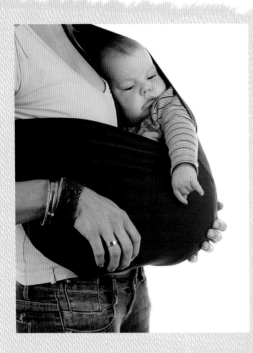

Fig.11 Not a good way of babywearing: huddled in one of the many pouches on the market.

Mei Tais

Special features
- *May* be used for almost all ages. The method of production and material quality determine this.

Bear in mind
- Not really suitable for newborns as the transverse pull is usually missing in the back area and so there is a lack of good support.

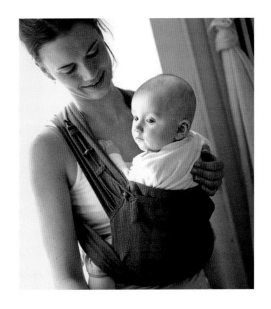

These traditional slings, originating in Asia, are sometimes referred to as the ancestor of the soft structured carrier. They originally consisted of a square piece of material used to carry the infant; the four corners are extended with straps. Two long straps are used as the shoulder straps and two as the hip belt. The quality of the material, and the width and style of the belts and straps determine the carrying quality. The simpler – and cheaper – the construction, the less suitable the Mei Tai is, particularly for smaller babies. This is because the principle does not provide any tension across the baby's back and thus there is no support in the back area. This can be offset by a good design and, in particular, the type of strap and the way it is fastend. A straight strap that only creates tension upwards (see Fig. 9, page 119) only provides minimum support to a baby's body. A weaving technique that is appropriate for a good wrap improves the carrying comfort and the support to the baby, if the design is suitable. Many mothers adapt their wraps to carriers of this type and today various manufacturers produce Mei Tais from good wrap materials.

Onbuhimos

Bear in mind

- Onbuhimos were originally intended for carrying babies on the back.
- Generally only suitable for older children who can already sit well.
- Suitability varies according to the type of manufacture and the material quality.
- Trying it out is essential.

At first glance, onbuhimos look like Mei Tais. Originally, however – and here descriptions and names become blurred nowadays – they did not have a hip belt and the straps only ran from the shoulder area of the child across the shoulders of the parent to the child's legs – like the shoulder straps on a rucksack. Many onbuhimos are even unsuitable for an older baby if his arms cannot be positioned above the shoulder straps due to a lack of height. In this situation the upper edge of the material of the pouch could be too tight around the child's neck and the head would thus fall backwards and force an awkward back position. You can see how important it is to try out all these carrying options.

Miscellaneous

There are many types of baby carrier, some of them very imaginative in design, which can help parents carry their baby. Whether or not they are suitable, and for which age of baby, must be thoroughly tested. Even an experienced babywearer can't always identify the 'snags' of each carrier system immediately, as some problems only become apparent as the baby gets older. The question then is: is this carrier so practical that it's worth spending money on a product you may only use for a short time? As always, the position of the child should also be checked. But think about yourself, too. Some much-lauded carriers may become torture for you after a long period of use. Every year manufacturers offer new models for lateral carrying (often simply called hip seats), which consist of some sort of seat for the child and a carrying harness that runs across the back and chest of the parent. Frequently the only adjustment that can be made is in the length of this carrying harness, so it can be adjusted to suit the person carrying, but not the child being carried. Such carriers are not suitable even for older children with a secure posture – who are often hardly supported at all. And they are no good for parents, as the pressure on just one shoulder is uncomfortable.

Ill thought-out product designs

At this point I would like to look at products available on the internet that are mostly pre-manufactured and have minimum adjustment options to suit the changing physical characteristics of babies. Accidents caused by babies falling out of badly designed pouches or 'sling-style infant carriers' have been known in the USA for years. With products of this type, which are often painstakingly manufactured and sold by enthusiastic and committed parents on their own, the focus is on the practical aspects. The specific anatomical characteristics of the infant, which are less familiar to a parent–manufacturer and which are – mostly – the be all and end all in manufacturing in the European regions, are widely neglected.

In addition, carrying in a lying position in particular is promoted in the USA, although babies carried in some products of this type are hunched up in such a way that the child's chin is pressed onto the chest (chin-to-chest position) and the airways are obstructed. In these cases, the fears of the child getting an inadequate oxygen supply are valid. But even large companies do not necessarily offer better adjusted or well thought-out product designs. The ill thought-out design of the voluminous bag-like pouch that hangs in front of the parent's stomach, which was offered by various manufacturers (bag-style slings, or sling-style infant carriers) causes accidents with dramatic consequences. In these pouches, which parents must hang over their shoulders and back, babies are carried in a *lying position*. However, this has caused the death of babies aged just a few weeks old, or who were sick, as their faces were pressed into the material. Additionally, the parents could not observe their children in these 'carrying bags'. Even though this product series was taken off the American–Canadian market in 2010 (see the corresponding web pages[99]), similar or equally unsuitable carriers continue to be launched onto the market. In a discussion group an American manufacturer asked which investigations really proved that the spine of a baby would not have the adult-typical S-shape.[100] This clearly shows the unsatisfactory background knowledge and quality of discussion in general of the industry, yet manufacturers are still making and selling such products.

Carrying the child facing outward

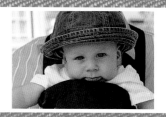

The advert shows young, modern and trendy parents carrying their little ones facing outwards. Beaming parents, smiling and active bundles of joy – there can't be anything wrong with this, can there? And yet, these babies are sitting in carriers 'back to front', in both senses of that expression.

Facing outwards – also called 'forward facing out' (FFO) – the positives of babywearing are thwarted:

1. The legs hang down, which does not encourage the healthy development of the hip joints.
2. The child cannot turn away from environmental stimuli of its own accord – they are forced to encounter all stimuli.
3. The child cannot observe the facial expressions of the parent, for information or an assessment of the situation, through a reassuring look.
4. Important physical contact is reduced to the relatively small back area of the baby,

which also has comparatively few tactile receptors.

There is no doubt that the still cartilaginous structures in the hip joint can be damaged during their development by enforced stretching. The construction of carriers designed so that infants face away from the parents often reinforces this stretching. As the baby does not sit in the carrier and instead more or less hangs on the crosspiece between the legs, the weight of the child is transferred to the still cartilaginous structures of the symphysis of the pelvis, and the testicles and the pubic area are also placed under more pressure – which they are not designed for.

Depending on the carrier, the shoulder straps also pull from the front over the child's shoulders back to the shoulder area of the adult. This means that the baby's shoulders are pushed backwards, which forces a stronger upright position of the upper body. Together with the hanging legs, this supports a hollow back.

Babies are carried facing outwards because parents want to offer more stimulation. A baby turned away from the adult in an upright, open body position is exposed to the environment and is often exceedingly agile. To the joy of the parents the multitude of impressions appear to enthuse their little one.

In this position, a baby is constantly exposed to the most diverse of stimuli without the opportunity to turn away when it is too much for him. As adults we have learned to differentiate between important and unimportant impressions and we have the corresponding experience and ability to blank out signals. However, a child must learn these. An oversupply of stimuli is and remains an oversupply, which must ultimately be worked through, often in the evening. In addition, not all stimulation is good stimulation. In this

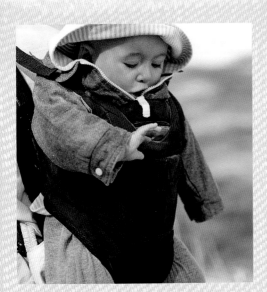

Fig. 12 Carrying the wrong way round: the legs are hanging down, the shoulders are pushed back – no eye contact is possible.

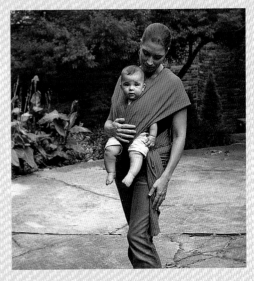

Fig. 13. Carrying the wrong way round: here it is especially clear that the child doesn't *sit* in the carrier, he is *hanging* in it.

position, babies lack the explanation they can gain from a reassuring glance at the face of the parent carrying him.

A strong visual representation can fascinate and captivate a child so that he can no longer withdraw, even if he is overstretched. The parents must then help the child. However, as they cannot observe the child's facial expressions with this carrying method and, if necessary, understand when their child needs support and protection, they cannot react.

Even resourceful babywearers haven't developed any tying options with the baby positioned the other way round in a wrap (see Fig. 13 page 171). To avoid a stretched leg position, some parents prefer the so-called **'Buddha carrying method'.** The baby sits huddled up in an Indian-style seated position in a wrap or ring sling and the legs and feet are packed inside. However, the legs are often very spread in this position and squeezed to the body, which causes adverse pressure on the hip socket and unsuitable orientation of the femoral head. At the same time, the feet are in an unnatural position and also fixed. **Overall, this carrying method is not recommended and certainly a child should not be carried in this position for a long period of time.**

It is likely that a carrier of this type will not cause any permanent damage when used for five or ten minutes, but there are better ways to satisfy a child's curiosity. Carrying on the hip or on the back in such a way that the active little one can look out over your shoulder are both suitable alternatives.

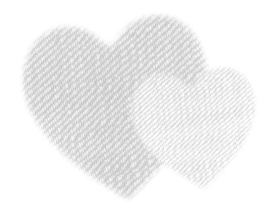

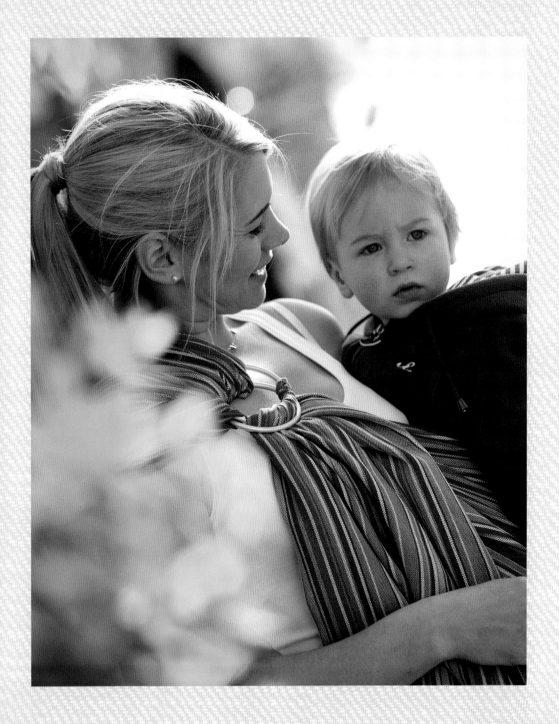

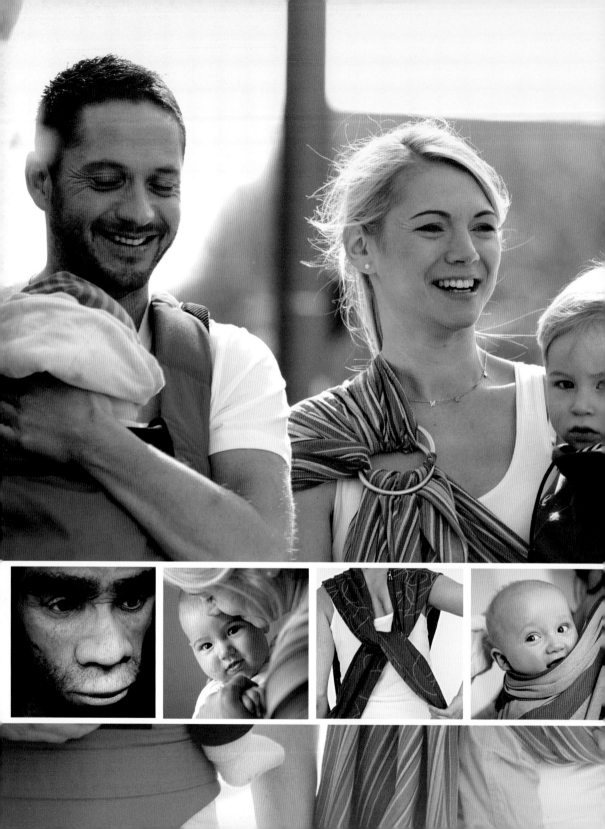

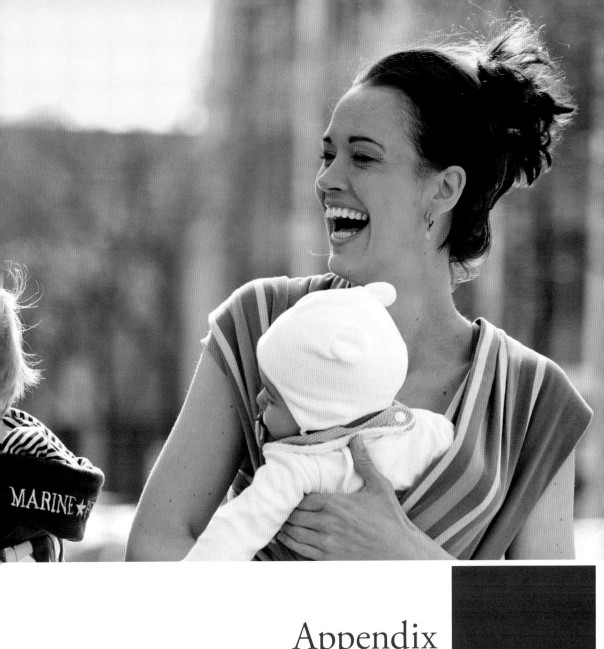

Appendix

Thanks

I would like to thank all the children and parents who, over many years, have been willing to provide me with varied information on the subject of carrying. I refer to those who allowed me to spend many hours observing them in their own homes, who were willing to sacrifice time answering difficult questionnaires, participating in interviews and answering many enquiries on the most diverse of subject areas, and who made themselves and their babies available to me to test out the different carriers and ways of tying them. Without them, this book would not have been possible.

On the selection of photos

Various companies provided material for the pictures in this book. For reasons of equality, after consultation, the publishers decided to avoid naming manufacturers and/or using logos for the products. We would like to sincerely thank the following companies for their friendly and generous support: Babylonia, ByKay, Didymos, Easycare, ERGObaby, Hoppediz and Storchenwiege. The selection of products shown was basically made by the babies, who energetically decided which of the images worked – and which didn't. Additional photographs by Shutterstock.

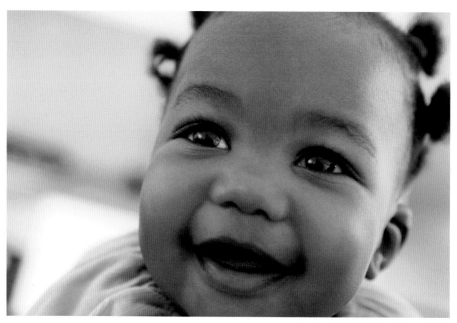

References

1. Heimerdinger, Timo: "Verwickelt aber tragfähig – Europäisch-ethnologischer Perspektiven auf ein Stück Stoff: das Babytragetuch". In: *Österreichische Zeitschrift für Volkskunde,* LXV/114 (3), 2011, S. 311–445

2. Hassenstein, Bernhard: *Verhaltens-biologie des Kindes.* Verlagshaus Monsenstein und Vannerdat, Münster 2007

3. Eliot, Lise: *Was geht da drinnen vor?* Berlin Verlag, Berlin 2010/Eliot, Lise: *What's Going on in There?* Bantam book, New York, Toronto, London, Sydney, Auckland, 1999

   Oerter, Rolf/Montada, Leo: *Entwicklungspsychologie.* Beltz, Weinheim 2002

4. Lovejoy, C. Owen/Suwa, Gen/Simpson, Scott W./Matternes, Jay H./White, Tim D.: "The Great Divides: Ardipithecus ramidus Reveals the Postcrania of Our Last Common Ancestors with African Apes". In: *Science,* Band 326, 2009

   Schwartz, Jeffrey H./Tattersall, Ian: "Fossil evidence for the origin of Homo sapiens". In: *American Journal of Physical Anthropology,* Band 143, Supplement 51, 2010, S. 94–121

   Wood, Bernhard/Harrison, Terry: "The evolutionary context of the first hominins". In: *Nature* 470, 2001, S. 347–352

5. Eibl-Eibesfeld, Irenäus: *Biologie des menschlichen Verhaltens: Grundriss der Humanethologie.* Blank, Berlin 2004/Eibl-Eibesfeld, Irenäus: *Human Ethology.* Aldine de Gruyter, New York 2008

   Medicus, Gerhard: *Was uns Menschen verbindet – Humanetholo-gische Angebote zur Verständigung zwischen Leib- und Seelenwissenschaften.* VWB, Berlin 2012

6. See reference 4.

7. I would like to thank Prof. Lang, Sempach, Switzerland, for permission to use the image of Goma, the first baby gorilla born in Basel Zoo.

8. Kirkilionis, Evelin: "Das Tragen des Säuglings im Hüftsitz – eine spezielle Anpassung des menschlichen Traglings". In: *Zoologische Jahrbücher,* 96, 1992, S. 395–415

   Kirkilionis, Evelin: *Der menschliche Säugling als Tragling unter besonderer Berücksichtigung der Prophylaxe gegen Hüftdysplasie,* Dissertation, Albert-Ludwigs-Universität Freiburg 1989

9. Staudach A: *Fetale Anatomie im Ultraschall.* Springer, Berlin 1986
   Bowermann RA: *Atlas of normal fetal*

ultrasonographic anatomy. Mosby, St. Louis, 1992

Sohn, Christof; Holzgreve, Wolfgang; Tercanli Sevgi: *Ultraschall in der Gynäkologie und Geburtshilfe.* Thieme Georg, Stuttgart, 2003.

Rohen, Johannes W./Yokochi, Chihiro/Lütjen-Drecoll, Elke: *Color Atlas of Anatomy: A Photographic Study of the Human Body.* Schattauer, Wolters Kluwer, Lippincott Williams & Wilkins, Philadelphia, Baltimor, New York, London, Buenos Aires, Hong Kong, Sydney, Tokyo, 2010

10. Debrunner, Hans U./Hepp, Wolfgang Rüdiger: *Orthopädisches Diagnostikum.* Thieme, Stuttgart, 2004

Osche, Günther: "Zur Evolutions-biologie des Menschen – Historische Aspekte der menschlichen Anatomie". In: Benninghoff, Alfred/Goertler, Kurt (Hrsg.): *Lehrbuch der Anatomie des Menschen. Makroskopische und mikroskopische Anatomie unter funktionellen Gesichtspunkten, Bd. 1.* Urban & Schwarzenberg, München, Berlin, Wien, 1975, S. 3–17

11. The drawings are based on photos or drawings of the books Sohn et al (2003), Rohen et al (2010) (see reference 9) and Schünke, Michael/ Schulte Erik/Schumacher, Udo: *Atlas of anatomy – General anatomy and musculoskeletal system.* Thieme, Stuttgart, New York, 2006.

12. See reference 8

13. Büschelberger, Johannes: "Ätiologie, Prophylaxe und Frühbehandlung der Luxationshüfte". In: *Beiträge zur Orthopädie und Traumatologie,* 11, 1964, S. 535–548

Büschelberger, Johannes: *Untersuch-ungen über Eigenart des Hüftgelenks im Säuglingsalter und ihre Bedeutung für die Pathogenese, Prophylaxe und Therapie der Luxationshüfte,* Postdoc-toral thesis, Dresden 1961

14. See reference 8

15. Fettweis, Ewald: *Hüftdysplasie: Sinnvolle Hilfe für Babyhüften.* Trias, Stuttgart 2004

Graf, Reinhard: *Sonographie der Säuglingshüfte und therapeutische Konsequenzen.* Thieme, Stuttgart 2009

Niethard, Fritz U.: *Kinder-orthopädie.* Thieme, Stuttgart, 2009

Pschyrembel, Willibald: *Klinisches Wörterbuch.* De Gruyter, Berlin 2012

Wülker, Nikolaus (Hrsg.): *Orthopädie und Unfallchirurgie.* Thieme, Stuttgart 2005

16. Fettweis 2004, see reference 15

17. Büschelberger 1961, see reference 13

18. Fettweis 2004, see reference 15

Fettweis, Ewald: "Über das Tragen von Babys und Kleinkindern in

Tüchern oder Tragehilfen". In: *Orthopädische Paxis,* 46 (2), 2010, S. 53–58

19. See reference 15 and Fettweis 2010, see reference 18

20. Au, Roland: *Ethnische Unterschiede im Transport von Säuglingen und Kleinkindern im Hinblick auf die Problematik der Hüftgelenkluxation,* Dissertation – Medizin (Charité), Humboldt-Universität Berlin 1969

    Palmen, Kurt: "Preluxation of the hip joint. Diagnosis and dislocation of the hip joint in Sweden during the years 1948–1960". In: *Acta Paediatrica,* 50, Supl. 129, 1961

    Palmen, Kurt: "Prevention of congenital dislocation of the hip. The Swedish experience of neonatal treatment of hip joint instability". In: *Acta orthopaedica scandinavica,* 55, Supl. 208, 1984, S. 1–107

21. Salter, Robert B.: "Etiology, pathogenesis and possible prevention of congenital dislocation of hip". In: *The Canadian Medical Association Journal,* 98(20), 1968, S. 933–945

22. Demuth, Carolin/Keller, Heidi/Yovsi, Relindis D.: "Cultural models in communication with infants: Lessons from Kikaikelaki, Cameroon and Muenster, Germany." In: *Journal of early childhood research,* 10, 2012, S. 70–87

    Keller, Heidi/Yovsi, Relindis D./Voelker, Susanne: "The role of motor stimulation in parental ethnotheories: The case of Camoroonian Nso and German women." In: *Journal of cross-cultural psychology,* 33, 2002, S. 398–414

23. Nagura, Shigeo: "Angeborene Hüftverrenkung und Volksgewohnheit" (zugleich Beitrag zur Kenntnis der sogenannten 'Dysplasie' der Pfanne bei angeborener Hüftverrenkung). In: *Zentralblatt für Chirurgie,* 24, 1940, S. 1042–1050

24. Fettweis 2004, see reference 15

25. Fettweis 2004, see reference 15

26. Fettweis 2004, see reference 15

27. Fettweis, Ewald: "Das kindliche Hüftluxationsleiden". In: Stahl, Christoph (Hrsg.): *Fortschritte in Orthopädie und Traumatologie,* Bd. 3, ecomed Fachverlag, Landsberg/Lech 1992

    Niethard 2009 as well as Pschyrembel 2012, see reference 15

28. Kirkilionis 1989, see reference 8

    Kirkilionis, Evelin: "Die Grundbedürfnisse des Säuglings und deren medizinische Aspekte – dargestellt und charakterisiert am Jungentypus

Tragling", Teil 2. In: *Notabene medici,* 2, 1997, S. 117–121

29. Kirkilionis 1989 and 1997, see reference 8 and 28

30. Au 1969, see reference 20

    Büschelberger, Johannes: "Das Dyadetuch: eine Möglichkeit zur Wiederherstellung des biologisch vorgegebenen Verhaltens bei der Pflege von Neugeborenen, Säuglingen und Kleinstkindern". In: *Kinderärztliche Praxis*, 11, 1981, S. 572–580

    Büschelberger 1964, see reference 13

    Nagura 1940, see reference 23

31. Zukunft, Barbara: *Moderne Säuglingsgymnastik.* Thieme, Stuttgart 1982

32. Kirkilionis, Evelin: unpublished data

    Kirkilionis, Evelin: "Vorteile zum Tragen kommen lassen". In: *Hebammenforum*, 14, 2013, S. 6–9

33. see reference 32 as well as reference 8 und 28

34. Kavruk, Hilal: *Der Einfluss des Tragens von Säuglingen und Kleinkindern in Tragehilfen auf die Entwicklung von Haltungsschäden im Schulkindalter – Untersuchungen mit der MediMouse®,* Dissertation, Universität Köln, 2010.

35. see reference 8 and 32

36. Stening, Waltraud/Nitsch, Patrizia/ Kribs, A./Weiß, R./Fricke, L./ Wassmer, G./Roth, B.: *Beobachtung der Vitalparameter früh- und reifgeborener Kinder während des Tragens in Tragehilfen.* Poster Kinderärztekongress München, 1999

    Stening, Waltraud/Nitsch, Patrizia/ Wassmer, Gernot/Roth, Bernhard: "Cardiorespiratory stability of premature and term infants carried in infant slings". In: *Pediatrics,* 110 (5), 2002

37. Anderson, Gene C.: "Touch and the kangaroo care method". In: Field, Tiffany M. (Hrsg.): *Touch in early development.* Lawrence Erlbaum, Hillsdale/NJ 1995, S. 35–51

    Marshall H. Klaus, John H Kennell, Phyllis H. Klaus: *Bonding: Building the foundations of secure attachment and independence.* Merloyd Lawrence book, Addison-Wesley Publishing Company, Inc. New York, 1995

    Ludington-Hoe, Susan M./Golant, Susan K.: *Kangaroo Care. The best you can do to help your preterm infant.* Bantam Books, 1993

    Strobel, Kornelia: *Frühgeborene brauchen Liebe. Was Eltern für ihr "Frühchen" tun können.* Kösel-Verlag, München 1998

38. Haug-Schnabel, Gabriele: "Der kompetente Säugling – das Verhaltensrepertoire im 1. Jahr". In: Wessel, Karl-Friedrich/Naumann, Frank (Hrsg.): *Kommunikation und Hu-*

manontogenese. Berliner Studien zur Wissenschaftsphilosophie & Humanontogenetik, Bd. 6, Kleine, Bielefeld 1994, S. 275–284

Schleid, Margret: "Die humanethologische Perspektive". In: Keller, Heidi (Hrsg.): *Handbuch der Kleinkindforschung*. Hans Huber, Bern, Göttingen, Toronto, Seattle 1997

39. Portmann, Adolf: *Biologische Fragmente zu einer Lehre vom Menschen*. Schwabe & Co., Basel 1969

40. Portmann 1969, see reference 39

41. Hassenstein, Bernhard: "Tierjunges und Menschenkind im Blick der vergleichenden Verhaltensforschung." In: *Berichte des Naturwissenschaftlich-Medizinischen Vereins in Innsbruck*, Bd. 58, 1970, S. 35–50

Hassenstein 2007, see reference 2

42. Hassenstein 2007, see reference 2

Masaracchia, Regina: *Gestillte Bedürfnisse*. Oesch Verlag, Zürich 2007

Weigert, Vivian: *Stillen: Das Begleitbuch für eine glückliche Stillzeit*. Kösel-Verlag, München 2010

La Leche League International: *The Womanly Art of Breastfeeding*. Pinter & Martin, London 2009

43. Pisacane, Alfredo/Continisio, Paola/Filosa, Cristina/Tagliamonte, Valeria/Continisio, Grazia I.: "Use of baby carriers to increase breastfeeding duration among term infants: the effects of an educational intervention in Italy". In: *Acta Paediatrica*, 101, 2012, S. 434–438

44. Hunziker Urs A., Barr R. B.: "Increased carrying reduces infant crying: A randomized controlled trial". *Pediatrics* 77(5), 1986, 641–648

Esposito, Gianluca/Yoshida, Sachine/Ohnishi, Ryuko/Tsuneoka, Yousuke/Rostagno, Maria del Carmen/Yokota, Susumu/Okabe, Shota/Kamiya, Kazusaku/Hoshino, Mikio/Shimizu, Masaki/Venuti, Paola/Kikusui, Takefumi/Kato, Tadafumi/Kuroda, Kumi O.: "Infant calming responses during maternal carrying in humans and mice". *Current Biology*, 23(9), 2013, 739-745

45. Kirkilionis, Evelin: unpublished data

46. Leon, Michael: "Touch and smell". In: Field, Tiffany M. (Hrsg.): *Touch in early development*. Lawrence Erlbaum, Hillsdale/NJ 1995, S. 81–87

47. Mizuno K./Mizuno N./Shinohara T./Noda, M.: "Mother-infant skin-to-skin contact after delivery results in early recognition of own mother's milk odour". In: *Acta Paediatrica*, 93 (12), 2004, S. 1640–1645

Moore Elizabeth R./Anderson Gene C./Bergman Nils/Dowswell, Therese:

"Early skin-to-skin contact for mothers and their healthy newborn infants". In: *The Cochrane Library*, published online: 16. Mai 2012

48. Ackermann, Diana: *Die schöne Welt der Sinne.* Europa Verlag, Hamburg, Wien, 2002/Ackermann, Diana: *A Natural History of the Senses.* Random House, New York, Toronto, 1995

    Field, Tiffany M./Schanberg, Saul M./Scafidi, Frank/Bower, Charles R./Vega-Lahr, Nitza/Garcia, R./Nystrom, Jerome/Kuhn, Cynthia M.: "Tactile/kinesthetic stimulation effects on preterm neonates". In: *Pediatrics*, 77, 1986, S. 654–658

    Scafidi, Frank A./Field, Tiffany M./Schanberg, Saul M./Bauer, Charles R./Tucci, Karen/Roberts, Jacqueline/Morrow, Connie/Kuhn, Cynthia M.: "Massage stimulates growth in preterm infants: A replication". In: *Infant behavior and development*, 13, 1960, S. 167–188

49. See reference 48

    Kuhn, Cynthia M./Schanberg, Saul M./Field, Tiffany/Symanski, Robert/Zimmerman, Eugene/Scafidi, Frank A./Roberts, Jackie: "Tactile-kinesthetic stimulation effects on sympathetic and adrenocortical function in preterm infants". In: *Journal of pediatrics*, 119 (3), 1991, S. 434–440

50. Ackerman 2002, see reference 48

    Cigale, Maricel/Field, Tiffany/Lundy, Brenda/Cuadra, Anai/Hart, Sybil: "Massage enhances recovery from habituation in normal infants". In: *Infant Behavior and Development,* 20 (1), 1997, 29–34

    Erlandsson, Kerstin/Dsilna, Ann/Fagerberg, Ingegard/Christensson, Kyllike: "Skin-to-skin care with the father after cesarean birth and its effect on newborn crying and prefeeding behaviour". In: *Birth,* 34, 2007, S. 105–114

51. Moore et al. 2012, see reference 47

    Renz-Polster, Herbert: *Menschenkinder – Plädoyer für eine artgerechte Erziehung.* Kösel-Verlag, München 2011

52. Field, Tiffany M.: "Infant massage therapy". In: Field, Tiffany M. (Hrsg.): *Touch in early development.* Lawrence Erlbaum, Hillsdale/NJ 1995, S. 105–114

    Haug-Schnabel, Gabriele: *Sexualität ist kein Tabu.* Herder, Freiburg 1997

    Haug-Schnabel, Gabriele: "Was der Kopf über den Körper weiß". In: *ZeT,* 5, 2001, S. 6–9

53. Eliot 2010, see reference 3

    Spitzer, Manfred: *Nervenkitzel*

– *Neue Geschichten vom Gehirn.*
Suhrkamp, Frankfurt 2006

54. Elliott, M. Ruth/Fisher, Kimberly/
Ames Elinor W.: "The effects of
rocking on the state and respiration of
normal and excessive cryers",
Canadian Journal of Psychology, 42 (2),
1988, S. 163–172
    Korner, A. F.: "Maternal rhythms
and waterbeds". In: Thoman, E.B.
(Hrsg.): *Origins of the infant's social
responsivness.* Lawrence Erlbaum
Association, Hillsdale/NJ 1979
    Korner, A. F./Thoman, E. B.: "The
relative efficacy of contact and
vestibular-proprioceptive stimulation
in soothing neonates", *Child development,* 43, 1972, S. 443–453
    Kramer, Lloyd I./Pierpont, Mary E.:
"Rocking waterbeds and auditory
stimuli to enhance growth of preterm
infants", *Journal of pediatrics,* 88 (2),
1976, S. 297–299

55. see reference 54

56. Ayres, Jean: *Bausteine der kindlichen
Entwicklung: Sensorische Integration
verstehen und anwenden.* Springer,
Berlin, 2013/Ayres, Jean: *Sensory
Integration and the Child: Understand-
ing hidden sensory challenges,* Western
Psychological Services, 2005
    Doering, Waltraut/Doering,
Winfried: *Sensorische Integration,*
*Anwendungsbereiche und Vergleich mit
anderen Fördermethoden/Konzepten.*
Borgmann, Dortmund 1996
    Keller, Heidi: *Handbuch der
Kleinkindforschung.* Verlag Hans
Huber, Bern 2003

57. Zimmer, Dieter E.: *Experimente des
Lebens.* Haffmans Verlag, Zürich 1989

58. Pellegrini A. D./Schmith, P. K.:
"Physical activity play: the nature and
function of a neglected aspect of
playing". In: *Child Development,* 1998
(3), S. 577–598
    Renz-Polster 2011, see reference 51
    Weber, Andreas: *Zurück auf die
Bäume,* Geo, 8, 2010

59. Eliot 2010, see reference 3
    Spitzer 2006, see reference 53

60. Clark, D. L./Kreutzberg, J./Chee, F.:
"Vestibular stimulation influence on
motor development in infants". In:
Science, 196, 1977, S. 1228–1229

61. Clark et al. 1977, see reference 60
    Adolph, Karen E./Karasik (Vishne-
vetsky), Lana B./Tamis-LeMonda,
Catherine S.: "Moving between
cultures: Cross-cultural research on
motor development." In: Bornstein,
Marc H. (Hrsg.): *Handbook of
cross-cultural developmental science, Vol.
1, Domains of development across
cultures.* New York 2010, S. 61–88
    Keller et al. 2002, see reference 22

Keller, Heidi: *Kinderalltag. Kulturen der Kindheit und ihre Bedeutung für Bindung, Bildung und Erziehung.* Springer-Verlag, Berlin 2011

62. Eliot 2010, see reference 3

63. See reference 56 as well as Eliot 2010, see reference 3

Ornitz, Edwald M.: "Normal and pathological maturation of vestibular function in the human child". In: Romand, R. (Hrsg): *Development of auditory and vestibular system,* Bd. 1, 1983, Academic Press, New York, S. 479–536

64. Grossmann, Karin/Grossmann, Klaus E.: *Bindung – das Gefüge psychischer Sicherheit.* Klett-Cotta, Stuttgart 2012

Kirkilionis, Evelin: *Bindung stärkt.* Kösel-Verlag, München 2008

65. See reference 64

66. Grossmann/Grossmann 2012, see reference 64

67. Guóth-Gumberger M./Hormann E: *Stillen.* Gräfe und Unzer, München 2004

Klaus et al. 1997, see reference 37

68. Erlandsson et al. 2007, see reference 50

69. Anisfeld, Elizabeth/Casper, Virginia/Nozyce, Molly/Cunningham, Nicholas: "Does infant carrying promote attachment? An experimental study of the effects of increased physical contact on the development of attachment". In: *Child development,* 61, 1990, S. 1617–1627

70. Anderson 1995, see reference 37

71. See reference 43

72. Palazzi, Stefano: "Die Motorik des Neugeborenen". In: *Die Umschau,* 84 (2), 1984, S. 50–84

73. Fredrickson, W. Timm/Brown, Josephine V.: "Posture as a determinant of visual behavior in newborns". In: *Child Development,* 46, 1975, S. 579–582

Zimmer, Katharina: "Die Schule der Sinne". In: *Geo Wissen – Kindheit und Jugend,* (2), September 1993, S. 36–39

74. Liedloff, Jean: *The Continuum Concept: In Search Of Happiness Lost,* Merloyd Lawrence, 1986

75. Papousek, Mechthild/Papousek, Hanus: "Intuitive elterliche Früherziehung in der vorsprachlichen Kommunikation. I. Teil: Grundlagen und Verhaltensrepertoire". In: *Sozialpädiatrie in Praxis und Klinik,* 12 (7), 1990, S. 521–527

76. See reference 64

77. See reference 64

Ainsworth, Mary D. S./Blehar, M.C./Waters, E./Wall, S.: "Patterns of attachment. A psychological study of the strange situation". In: Erlbaum, Hillsdale/NJ 1978.

Ainsworth, Mary D. S.: "Patterns of attachment". In: *The Clinical Psychologist*, 38 (2), 1985, S. 27–29

78. Schieche, Michael/Spangler, Gottfried: "Individual differences in biobehavioral organization during problem-solving in toddlers: The influence of maternal behavior, infant-mother attachment, and behavioral inhibition on the attachment-exploration balance". In: *Developmental Psychobiology* 46 (4), 2005, S. 293–306

Spitzer, Manfred: *Medizin für die Bildung: Ein Weg aus der Krise.* Spektrum Akademischer Verlag, Heidelberg 2010

79. See reference 64 as well as Schieche/ Spangler 2005, see reference 78

Spangler, Gottfried: "Die Rolle kindlicher Verhaltensdispositionen für die Bindungsentwicklung". In: Spangler, Gottfried/Zimmermann, Peter (Hrsg.): *Die Bindungstheorie. Grundlagen, Forschung und Anwendung.* Klett-Cotta, Stuttgart 1995, S. 178–190

Stephan, Christine: "Bindungsbeziehung – Spielbeziehung – Kompetenzentwicklung". In:

Spangler, Gottfried/Zimmermann, Peter (Hrsg.): *Die Bindungstheorie. Grundlagen, Forschung und Anwendung.* Klett-Cotta, Stuttgart 1995, S. 265–280

80. Konner, Melvin J.: Relations Among Infants and Juveniles in Comparative Perspective. In: Lewis, M.; Rosenblum, L. A. (eds.): *The Origins of Behavior, Vol. 4: Friendship and peer relations.* New York, London, Sydney, Toronto, John Wiley & Sons, 1975, S. 99-129

Konner, Melvin J.: "Maternal care, infant behavior and development among the !Kung". In: Lee, Richard B./de Vore, Irven. (Publ.): *Kalahari hunter-gatherers. Studies of the !Kung San and their neighbors.* University Press, Cambridge, Massachusetts 1976/1999, S. 218–245

Renz-Polster 2011, see reference 51

Schiefenhövel, Wulf: "Bindung und Loslösung – Sozialisationspraktiken im Hochland von Neuguinea". In: Eggers, Christian (Hrsg.): *Bindung und Besitzdenken beim Kleinkind.* Urban & Schwarzenberg, München, Wien, Baltimore 1984

81. Konner 1975 and 1976, see reference 80

82. Rosenfeld, A. A./Wissen N.: *The*

over-scheduled child: avoiding the hyper-parenting trap. Griffin 2000

83. Bensel, Joachim: *Wie Sie Ihr Schreibaby verstehen und beruhigen. Entlastung für Eltern – Beruhigung fürs Baby.* ObersteBrink, Ratingen 2003

    Konner, 1975 and 1976, see reference 80

    Sears, William, Sears, Martha: *The attachment parenting book. A common-sense guide to understanding and nurturing your baby.* Boston, Little, Brown and Company, 2001

84. See reference 54

85. Ackerman 2002, see reference 48

86. Whitelaw, Andrew/Sleath, Katharine: "Myth of the marsupial mother: home care of very low birth weight babies in Bogota, Colombia". In: *The Lancet,* 325 (no 8439), 1985, S. 1206–1208

    Klaus et al. 1997, see reference 37

87. See reference 37

    Kuhn et al. 1991, see reference 49

88. Anderson 1995, see reference 37

    Feldman, R./Eidelman, A. I./Sirota, L./Weller, A.: "Comparison of skin-to-skin (kangaroo) and traditional care: Parenting outcomes and preterm infant development". In: *Pediatrics,* 110, 2002, S. 16–26

    Field, Tiffany: "Massage therapy facilitates weight gain in preterm infants". In: *Current Directions in Psychological Science,* 10, 2001, S. 51–54

89. Klaus, Marshall H.: "Touching during and after childbirth". In: Field, Tiffany M. (Hrsg.): *Touch in early development.* Lawrence Erlbaum, Hillsdale/NJ 1995, S. 19–33

    Klaus et al. 1997, see reference 37

    de Leeuw, R: "De Kangoeroemethode". In: *Nederlands Tijdschrift voor Geneeskunde,* 131 (34), 1987, S. 1484–1487

90. Marcovich, Marina/de Jong, Theresia M.: *Frühgeborene – zu klein zum Leben?* Kösel-Verlag, München 2008

91. Honigmann, Klaus: *Lippen- und Gaumenspalten.* Huber, Bern 1998

    Masaracchia, Regina: *Gespaltene Gefühle. Lippen-, Kiefer-, Gaumenspalten.* Oesch Verlag, Zürich 2007

    Naumann, Sandra: *Frühförderung bei Kindern mit Lippen-Kiefer-Gaumen-Sebel-Fehlbildung.* Schulz-Kirchner Verlag, Idstein 2010

92. Lehmann, Siri: "Tragen – Für einen guten Start ins Leben". In: *Leben mit Down-Syndrom,* 63, 2010, S. 36–38

93. Prof. Hans-Michael Straßburg, Würzburg, personal communication

94. Bialocerkowski, Andrea E./Vladusic, Sharon L./Wei Ng Choong: "Prevalence, risk factors, and natural history

of positional plagiocephaly: a systematic review". In: *Developmental Medicine & Child Neurology*, 50 (8), 2008, S. 577-586

Renz-Polster, Herbert: *Tragen aus kinderärztlicher Sicht*, http://kinderverstehen.de/images/Tragen_Renz-Polster.pdf

95. see reference 32

96. Badinter, Elisabeth: *Der Konflikt. Die Frau und die Mutter*. C. H. Beck, München 2010.

Heimerdinger 2011, see reference 1

97. Davis, Beth E./Moon, Rachel Y./Sachs, Hari C./Ottolini, Mary C.: "Effects of sleep position on infant motor development". In: *Pediatrics* 102, 1998, S. 1135–1140.

Eliot 2010, see reference 3

98. www.verhaltensbiologie.com/forschen/tragen/Kirkilionis_Statement_Trage_Todesfaelle.pdf

www.cpsc.gov/cpscpub/prerel/prhtml10/10165.html

www.cpsc.gov/cpscpub/prerel/prhtml10/10177.html

Kirkilionis, Evelin: "Tragen ist nicht gleich Tragen". In: *Deutsche Hebammenzeitschrift*, 7, 2010, S. 58–61

99. See reference 98

100. Personal communication: Frome, Beate, 2012, Smithfield, Utah, USA

Image references

Photographs: Susanne Krauss
Ausnahmen: P. 22: Eric Gevaert/Fotolia.com; p. 26: Bastos/Fotolia.com; p. 29: With kind permission by Prof. Lang, Switzerland; p. 35: © Pakhnyushchyy/Fotolia.com; p. 38: evgenyatamanenko/Fotolia.com; p. 44: Petro Feketa/Fotolia.com; p. 46: thongsee/Fotolia.com; p. 47: Digitalpress/Fotolia.com; p. 49: NatesPics/iStockphoto; p. 60 and 93: Vitalinko/Fotolia.com; p. 74 and 97: Robert Emprechtinger/Fotolia.com; p. 90 and 91: Tobilander/Fotolia.com; p. 94: Joni Hofmann/Fotolia.com; p. 106/107 (large): Kati Molin_rf/shutterstock; p. 126/127 (background): mninni/Fotolia.com; p. 133: molka/iStockphoto; p. 168: ehrenberg-bilder/Fotolia.com; p. 170: Studio1One/iStockphoto; p. 171 rechts: kilahfunkadelic/iStockphoto; p. 171 links: trait2lumiere/iStockphoto, p. 12, p. 16, p.25, p. 35, p. 44, p. 100, p. 176 Shutterstock.
Fabric background: (for example p. 2/3 and p. 29): chaoss/Fotolia.com
Illustrations: p. 37, 119: Mascha Greune

The publishers would like to thank everyone who has contributed to the success of the photograph production, in particular: Susanne Krauss, Laura Bertoldi, our child and adult models, the Zentrum für Natürliche Geburt und Elternsein e.V. (Centre for Natural Birth and Parenting) in Munich, as well as Anja Jablonski–Sacher and 'Sepp'.

Index

kangaroos 23
knees above bottom position 50–1, 112 *see also* spread-
    squat leg posture
knee-to-knee support 112, 118–19, 142, 145
knots 126–7
Konner, Melvin J. 88
!Kung people 21, 88
kyphosis (slightly rounded spine) 35, 36

learning difficulties in older children, benefits of early
    carrying for 72
learning to carry
    getting tuition on tying methods 122
    timing of 102
legs hanging down position 118–19
legs-in vs legs-out 142
length of time carried (daily) 53–4, 99, 103, 110
Liedloff, Jean 84
low carrying 119
Lycra/ Spandex 130
lying-down carrying positions
    cradle carry 160–3
    many people insist on 53, 58
    not essential 53, 58, 86, 110
    potential dangers of 166, 169
    and pouches 166, 169

malformations (baby's) and the benefits of carrying 93
massage, benefits of 62–3
material used for woven wraps 129–30
Mei Tais 11, 128, 167
midwives, as source of advice 10, 98, 114, 128
Montagu, Ashley 66
motor development, babywearing encourages 71–2, 84
movement
    babywearing requires baby to move more 71–2, 95
    beneficial in cases of hip dysplasia 50
    children need to experience 68–9
    parental movement stimulates baby's proprio-
        vestibular senses 65–6
    rocking as calming 19, 20, 65
multisensory integration 67–9
muscle tone, carrying babies with poor 94–5

Nagura, Shigeo 46
nappies (diapers)
    accommodating in carriers 112
    double nappies ('broad diapering') 51
Neanderthals 26
neuro-processing 67
new situations - a carried baby is in the best position to
    explore 85–6
newborns
    back carries 155, 157

can be carried upright 53, 58, 86, 110
cradle carry 160–3
Mei Tais not suitable for 167
newborn inserts for soft-structured carriers 114
no need to have feet tucked in 142
ring slings not always suitable for 165
simple hip carry 149–50
stretchy wraps 130–1
nidiculous young 22
nidifugous young 22
North American Indians 40, 46

Old Anna 66
onbuhimos 11, 168
out of sight out of mind - babies can't understand absence
    17–18
over-stimulation, baby can turn away from 84, 150,
    170–1
oxygen supply 55, 160

pain whilst carrying (parental) 99–100, 114, 130
palmar grasp reflex 25
papooses 40
parent-child relationship 11, 74–89
parenting 'philosophy' 103
parents, benefits of babywearing for
    calming benefits of babywearing for mother 63
    easier to manage daily life 8, 74, 98–9
    with premature babies 91
    promotes secure bonding with baby 8, 62–3, 74–89,
        92
    reduced stress 74, 80
passive clinging young 23, 27
pelvis, position of
    adult's 28
    baby's 38, 40–1
perception, babies' 17–18
personality development 76
physical closeness, need for
    as babies' basic need 8–9, 15, 19
    babies have varying needs for 102–3, 110
    for babies with disabilities 93–5
    children with hip dysplasia still need 48
    as element of being 'active clinging young' 23
    needs to be positive for parents too 99–101
    other ways to provide 63, 101–2
    for premature babies 90–2
    reduced physical contact in forward facing out
        position 170
    and secure attachment 78–80, 82–3, 88–9
    and sensory development 60–9
picking up babies, biological basis for 17
plantar grasp reflex 130
pocket wrap cross carry (PWCC) 138

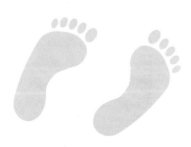